Restore Your Temple

Restore Your Temple

**7 LIFE-CHANGING STEPS TO REVIVE YOUR
SPIRITUAL, MENTAL, AND PHYSICAL HEALTH**

James Kinsella, MD

This book is dedicated to:
God who loves me, guides me, comforts me, forgives me, and
many times carries me.
Let Your will be done.

And to:
My amazing wife who I love more and more each day.

Table of Contents

Part I

RESTORE YOUR TEMPLE

Introduction

Do you not know that your bodies are temples of the Holy Spirit, who is in you, whom you have received from God? You are not your own; you were bought at a price. Therefore honor God with your bodies.
1 Corinthians 6:19–20

Does your body feel like a temple of the Holy Spirit? Do you honor God with the way you honor your body, mind, and soul? Many people treat their vehicles, homes, or other things in their lives with more care than they do their bodies. You would probably never even consider putting artificial fuel into your car if you knew it was bad for your gas mileage or the long-term health of your vehicle. Unfortunately, whether you know it or not, you are very likely doing this to your body and mind every day.

You are considering an intense, life-changing body, mind, and soul restoration plan. This is not just a book you will read; it is a way of life that will transform you. It is not a thirty-day cleanse. It is not a quick-fix diet. It will not be easy. Nothing worth doing ever is. Easy things bring little fulfillment.

Still, the concept of difficulty is relative. Living in poverty is difficult. Battling cancer is difficult. Broken relationships are difficult. Feeling sick and depressed is difficult. Chronic disease is difficult. So compared to those things, this will be easy.

3

The plan is going to take commitment, fortitude, and support. It is going to take prayer, guidance, and learning to lean on God. If you don't have those things or don't know how to do those things, you have even more reason to commit to this restoration plan immediately.

You were created with a purpose. You should be excited and full of anticipation about the potential of restoring your temple for yourself, your loved ones, and the God who created you for great things. Jesus paid a great price—you were bought for a price. There will be some financial and other costs associated with restoring your body, mind, and soul. However, this will not be as financially or emotionally expensive as treating diabetes, high blood pressure, autoimmune diseases, fibromyalgia, migraine, high cholesterol, fatty liver, osteoporosis, inflammatory bowel disease, irritable bowel syndrome, chronic constipation, ADD, mood disorders, Alzheimer's, or one of the many other diseases that I could list here, including multiple types of cancer. You are going to spend it now or pay for it later. There may be no better return on investment than investing now in your physical and spiritual health.

This moment is one you will remember. It is your chance to start honoring your body.

When I started the journey that led me to write this book, I was taking four very potent prescription medications that cost upwards of two to three hundred dollars per month. I was missing out on life and felt sick almost every minute of every day, mostly because of how I treated my mind and fed my body. I was less productive at work and was not the husband or dad I wanted to be. I was not able to do the work I knew the Lord had planned for me.

You may not even know what you are missing out on or know how it feels to have a restored temple. That may be the greatest price of *not* making this decision.

One final question: can you do this? Yes. You were made to do it. The cool thing about this complete restoration plan is that it is not just a quick-fix diet or exercise program. This is a heart, soul, and mind restoration program, in addition to a body and health restoration. So committing to this program and starting it will eventually give you the tools to complete it, and more important, stick with it.

Here is my promise to you: this will be worth it. You will gain control of your health, including your stamina and physical fitness. You will have improved relationships. You will have an overall sense of well-being and achievement. You will learn to find peace in the midst of stress and commotion. Best of all, you will learn to be in relationship with your loving God.

> He gives strength to the weary
>> and increases the power of the weak.
> Even youths grow tired and weary,
>> and young men stumble and fall;
> but those who hope in the Lord
>> will renew their strength.
> They will soar on wings like eagles;
>> they will run and not grow weary,
>> they will walk and not be faint. (Isaiah 40:29–31)

Okay. Here we go! Don't read on unless you are all in. This is your point of no return.

About Me

I am a follower and lover of Jesus Christ, who is my God, Father, Rock, Redeemer, Teacher, and Guide. He is the Truth and the Way. He is all God and all man. He is the great and holy I AM. He is the Alpha and the Omega. He paid the price for my sinful ways, and, maybe best of all, He wants to be my friend and loves me enough not to leave me where I am.

I am a husband to an amazing wife, Elissa, who loves me like Jesus does. I know this because she loves and cares for me even when I am not at my best. She supported me through sickness and great stress. She is a beautiful woman. On top of all this, my favorite thing about her is that she really loves Jesus and wants you to also.

I am a dad to three unbelievable, awesome kids: Devin, Jalyn, and Mason. They are all perfectly different from each other and are the kind of kids who make me proud (and honored) to say I am their dad. I could write a book about the life lessons I have learned from these wonderful blessings with whom God has entrusted me. Watching them grow is fun, exciting, scary, crazy, and sometimes like looking at my own life in a mirror. Most of all, it is inspiring to watch them grow in their love for God.

I am also a son, brother, uncle, cousin, and friend. I cherish all of these relationships.

I am a physician. I am also a seminary student pursuing a doctoral degree in ministry.

I am a long-suffering survivor of many health issues centering on what started as migraine headaches and transformed into chronic supraorbital neuralgia with allodynia. However, I believe this is a systemic disease with many other whole-body symptoms—so many that I will not try to list them. I was so sick just a few years ago that, in my mid-thirties, I was flat out denied disability insurance. I was not offered a higher rate or a plan with exceptions; I was denied.

This disease is in my case entirely caused, or at least greatly determined, by my interaction with my environment, primarily my diet and my internal reaction to stress. I always kind of knew this, but it took me twenty years to finally begin to put the pieces together. This struggle has been a very important part of my journey. It has kept me humble. It has forced me to be introspective. It has afforded me the time, desire, and need to turn to God for all parts of my life. This is a journey that I am still and will forever be on. It is also the reason that I have put so much of my time, attention, and pursuit of wisdom into restoring all the parts of my body, my temple. I didn't start this with the expectation that this would become a great passion of my life. I didn't start this thinking it would be a biblical study in restoration of the temple that the Lord has provided for my soul. I didn't think I would one day want to use the knowledge gained to lead others to live a life of health and fulfillment or to lead them toward Christ. The best part is God knew.

> For my thoughts are not your thoughts, neither are your ways my ways," declares the Lord. "As the heavens are higher than the earth, so are my ways higher than your ways and my thoughts than your thoughts. (Isaiah 55:8-9)

Outline: An Overview

Remember this is not a short-term change or a quick-fix diet. It is a life restoration plan. If your temple needs some work, this is your chance for comprehensive life change.

The Bible refers to Jesus as the Cornerstone. In the book of Matthew, Jesus said:

> *Therefore everyone who hears these words of mine and puts them into practice is like a wise man who built his house on the rock. The rain came down, the streams rose, and the winds blew and beat against that house; yet it did not fall, because it had its foundation on the rock.* (Matthew 7:24–27)

He is the foundation and the cornerstone. We should build our lives upon Him, so that when the winds blow, we will not fall. This temple restoration project is based upon this fundamental truth.

It is also based upon the fact that just changing one thing will not be sustainable or worth your time. The goal of this is not only to change your body and health but also to change your heart, soul, and mind. Jesus said we are supposed to *"Love the Lord your God with all your heart and with all your soul and with all your mind"* (Matthew 22:37). This life restoration plan will focus on improving all aspects of who you are, both physical and nonphysical.

The blueprints for restoring your temple come in seven parts. I will refer to them as the seven building blocks of the plan. It will take you at least seven weeks to begin to implement them. Part II of the book includes worksheets to walk you through these building blocks over seven weeks. Use these worksheets daily and have them with you, as a guide. And even at week seven you will not be finished; that moment will simply be the beginning of the rest of your life. Your temple will be restored to the point that you can begin to truly live in it.

This is a seven-week kickoff to a new way of living—a catalyst. Buckle up.

There will be some references to research and detailed explanation when deemed necessary for understanding. However, this is meant to be an easy read. Implementation is the key. I do not want you to get bogged down in the details. Multiple resources will be provided for those who want or need further explanation.

Here are the seven building blocks:

1. Prayer and Study: Prepare Your Soul and Mind
2. Diet: Fuel Your Body
3. Exercise: Strengthen Your Temple
4. Stress Reduction: Find Peace for Your Soul
5. Community: Choose Your Companions
6. Removing Toxins: Cleanse Your Life
7. Rest and Worship: Reset Your Compass

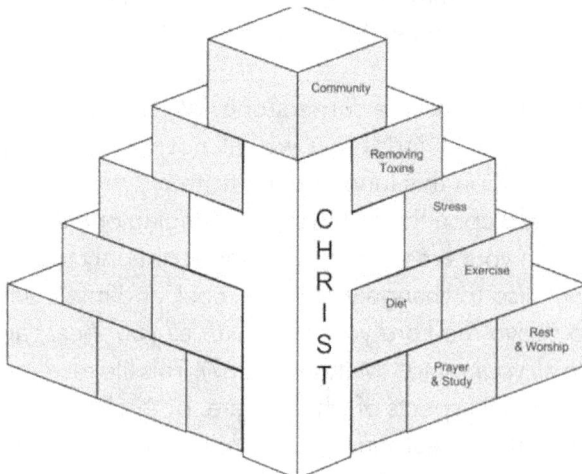

Each part will have:

- An explanation and some necessary details
- A step-wise plan for implementation into the seven-week restoration program in the weekly worksheets (Part II)
- Encouragements
- Tools
- Challenges

Demolition
(and Preparation) Week

For those of you who watch television shows involving home restoration, the projects always start with some demolition. The same holds true for this project. Think of this as a restoration project and your temple as a fixer-upper. Some walls are going to need to be knocked down, and some things are going to need to be thrown in the dumpster. We all have some parts of our lives that need to be taken down before we can begin to build them up. It is not always the best plan to build on the existing structure. Some of these structures will need to be completely rebuilt.

So for the first week (or more, if that's what it takes) you will be doing some demolition. You will also need some building supplies. In order to remodel or restore anything, some new pieces will need to be added.

Each building block will have its own demolition components or its own supplies, with a day dedicated to each. This part cannot be skipped. You should complete each part so that when you start this life-changing restoration project, there will be no roadblocks to your ultimate success. Also, make sure you obtain everything on the building supply list so you are prepared with what you need.

Let's look at each of the seven building blocks and the associated preparation and demolition. You will complete these over the next seven days.

Demolition Day 1

- Read Building Block 1.
- You will need a Bible (suggestion: New International Version).
- Download a Bible app (suggestion: Bible app from Lifechurch.tv).
- Plan a time for morning prayer (at least ten minutes).

Demolition Day 2

- Read Building Block 2.
- Download the MyFitnessPal app on your smartphone and learn how to use it. Track everything you eat and drink for at least three days this week before you start the seven-week restoration. This should be a normal eating week for you to give you an idea of what your food intake is like before starting this plan.
- On the tracking app we will pay most attention to added sugar content, carbohydrate totals, and dietary breakdown (percentage of calories from fat, protein, and carbs).
- Track the following each day:
  Carbs(g) _____ _____ _____ _____ _____
  Sugar (g) _____ _____ _____ _____ _____
  Fat % _____ _____ _____ _____ _____
- Use the MSG list to collect and quarantine any food, spice, or beverage with an ingredient on the list.
- Then collect and quarantine anything with sugar added (any food with greater than five grams per serving of sugar).
- Finally, do the same with any foods obviously containing gluten: wheat, wheat flour, rye, barley, and bran. This includes (but is not limited to) bread, waffles, bagels, and donuts.
- These three groups of food should be removed from your home at the end of demolition week, on the day prior to starting week one of the restoration plan. I suggest the garbage.
- Look at the included shopping list (appendix) and start to plan your shopping and prepare for week one.

Demolition Day 3

- Read Building Block 3.
- Begin to plan a good time to set aside thirty minutes to exercise three to six days per week.
- Plan where you are going to exercise. If it is in your home, prepare the space.
- Purchase any equipment you may need. A set of dumbbells may be all you need.
- Record your weight and any other measurements you would like to track here:
  Weight:_____
  Waist size:_____
  Other measurement(s):_____
- Do not weigh or measure yourself again until week five at the earliest (see worksheets).

Demolition Day 4

- Read Building Block 4.
- Purchase a simple journal or notebook.
- Plan a time for evening journaling (approximately ten minutes).
- Start thinking about ways to listen to Christian music (e.g., radio, Pandora, iTunes).
- Listen to *Lord, I Need You* by Matt Maher.

Demolition Day 5

- Read Building Block 5.
- Start thinking about how you spend your time.
- Learn the hierarchy of relationships.

Demolition Day 6

- Read Building Block 6.

Demolition Day 7

- Read Building Block 7.
- If you do not have a church or would like to try a new church, start thinking about this and do some research.
- Plan for your weekly day of rest.

Once you have finished these, you are ready to start! See the worksheets in Part II.

BUILDING BLOCK 1

Prayer and Study: Prepare Your Soul and Mind

> *The Lord is near to all who call on him,*
> *to all who call on him in truth.*
> PSALM *145:18*

You will not be able to do this on your own. The good news is that you were not made or meant to do this alone. The God who created you wants to be your Life Coach. He wants to be your friend. He is near to you if you will call on Him.

Have you ever done so? You may say that you believe in God and maybe even that you love Him, but does your life give example to this? Do you have a relationship with Him? If you stopped believing in God today would anyone notice?

So how do we as God's creation build a relationship with the amazing and awesome Creator? The answer to this is pretty straightforward. How do you build a loving relationship with anyone? You get to know them, spend time with them, and speak with them frequently. That is what this building block is all about.

A relationship with the God who loves you starts with prayer. If you really love Him or want to love Him, this is step number one. You cannot skip this building block and expect to restore your temple. Martin Luther once said, "To be a Christian without prayer is no more possible than to be alive without breathing."

James 4:8 says if you come near to God, He will draw near to you. This drawing close is the building of a relationship, a friendship, and your ability to trust and obey Him as your Father. We are to have a childlike confidence and carefree happiness because of our trusting relationship with Him. It is in your quiet time of prayer that you will cast your concerns on Him and begin to hear His guidance and advice to you through His still, small voice. This is the relationship He created you to have, the reason for your being.

Prayer

So you might be asking "How do I pray?" There are many resources to help with this, but I will give you a plan and a kick start to use for this initial seven weeks that will hopefully get you started on a lifelong, loving relationship with your awesome Creator.

Let's start with the instruction given by Jesus on the subject of how to pray.

> *This, then, is how you should pray:*
> *"Our Father in heaven,*
> *hallowed be your name,*
> *your kingdom come,*
> *your will be done,*
> *on earth as it is in heaven.*
> *Give us today our daily bread.*
> *And forgive us our debts,*
> *as we also have forgiven our debtors.*
> *And lead us not into temptation,*
> *but deliver us from the evil one. (Matthew 6:9–13)*

This is Jesus giving us an example to use of how to pray. So for this building block we can follow His lead. We will use the acronym ACTS as we pray each day. These four parts of prayer can be a guide for you as you start to begin each and every day with prayer.

ACTS of Prayer (How to Pray)

1. Adoration and Praise: "God, I adore you because you are . . ."
- Putting into words the gratitude we should have whenever we consider all that God has done for us.
- Thanking and praising God for who He is.

2. Confession: "God, I confess that I have . . ."
- *If we confess our sins, he is faithful and just and will forgive us our sins and purify us from all unrighteousness* (1 John 1:9).
- Be real with ourselves and with God about our shortcomings.
  - God won't answer our prayers when there is unconfessed sin in our lives.
  - God won't forgive us unless we forgive others (see Matthew 6:14–15).
  - Confession has an effect upon our physical health (see Psalm 32:3–7).
  - God is not against us because of our sin. He is with us against our sin.

3. Thanksgiving
- *Do not be anxious about anything, but in every situation, by prayer and petition, with thanksgiving, present your requests to God* (Philippians 4:6).
- Adoration vs. thanksgiving:
  - Adoration is thanking God for who He is.
  - Thanksgiving is thanking God for what He has done.
- We should give Him thanks in all things (see 1 Thessalonians 5:18).

4. Supplication (asking God to supply)
- Ask for personal requests. Especially:
  - Wisdom (see James 1:5–8)
  - Health (see 2 Corinthians 12:7–9)
  - Daily needs (see Matthew 6:33)
  - Resisting temptation (see Matthew 26:41)
- Pray for and present requests for others.

Here is an example of what an ACTS prayer might look like:

> God you are so awesome and good. I confess to you that I have fallen short. I have done _____ and ask for your forgiveness. Thank you for all you have done and continue to do for me. Specifically, I thank you for _____. Please give me your guidance and wisdom. Give me the strength and power I need to restore my temple. Please do _____ for me. For my family I ask that you _____. I love you Lord. Amen.

The other thing I would like you to add to this is silence. At the end of your time of prayer sit in silence for a few minutes. Listen. You have just asked God to guide you. Let Him. Feel His presence. When you pray, you are speaking directly to God. He is present. You are not speaking to Him as though He is off on some distant planet. He is near. He is with you.

Realizing He is right there with you is a powerful and very important part of prayer. When you realize this and begin to pray to Him in this way, something amazing happens. At the end of your prayers you feel His presence. You begin to hear and feel His response to you. A relationship forms. The relationship you were created to have. The relationship that will change everything.

When should you pray? The Bible says we should pray without ceasing. In other words we should go to God for everything. He should be and will be part of your daily walk. If you have issues with your vehicle, you take it to a mechanic. If you have issues with your tooth, you go to a dentist. If you want to know how to best live your life, go to the One who created you and life itself. Once you experience His presence and great power in your time of prayer, you will learn to go to Him throughout your day.

As part of this restoration plan you will start your day with dedicated prayer time. Wake up and give Him at least the first ten minutes of your day. For these ten minutes, you will use the ACTS acronym to learn to talk with your Creator. So you will wake up, find a quiet place, and start your day with a conversation with the Lord of the Universe. How awesome is that? I will walk you through this in the provided weekly worksheets.

Bible Study

The second part of this building block is study. God, in His grace and wisdom, has provided us with the instruction manual for life. The Bible is not just a group of stories or a piece of abstract literature. It is the Word of God in a form you can touch and feel. It is a gift from Him to you.

If you truly love Him or want to love Him, you should have a deep and longing desire to know what His instructions are for your life. Out of that will come a desire for obedience to His Word: *"Do not merely listen to the word, and so deceive yourselves. Do what it says."* (James 1:22).

You may have read the Bible and studied it thoroughly. You may have never opened the Bible. Regardless, God wants to speak into your life through His Word, and you will begin to do that in these seven weeks. A Bible and the Bible app were in your supply list. So, at this point you at the very least should have a Bible. Some good books of the Bible to start with are Proverbs, Mark, John, Matthew, Luke, and James.

I have supplied you with a seven-week reading plan that will focus primarily on the life of Jesus. This will be laid out for you in the weekly worksheets. I will provide specific readings for each week. If something comes up and you get behind, set aside a larger period of time one day and catch up. After each reading ask yourself these two questions:

1.   How would I summarize what I just read?
2.   What does it mean for me in my daily life?

Just starting with these two simple questions will unlock many truths from God's Word into your life. You will begin to see how relevant the Bible is and how God instructs us through it.

The Bible is God lovingly guiding us to true happiness, peace, and fulfillment. Who wouldn't want that? How many people do you know who actually have those things in their lives? You are about to. Get ready. He wants you to have a life of fulfillment: *"The thief comes only to steal and kill and destroy; I have come that they may have life, and have it to the full"* (John 10:10).

My challenge to you is to make this a priority in your life. Start each day getting to know Jesus. He wants to know you. He wants you to know

Him deeply. He also wants you to go to Him for everything, not just the big things. He is your Creator. He created life. If you want to know how to live and live well, He should be your ultimate guide.

You will use these building blocks to add some new habits to your life. These habits will become desires. You will begin to experience a life full of God's presence. You will begin to depend on Him, and He will not let you down. Jesus is the cornerstone of your temple, and with prayer and Bible study you are laying the foundation.

BUILDING BLOCK 2

Diet: Fuel Your Body

So whether you eat or drink or whatever
you do, do it all for the glory of God.
1 CORINTHIANS 10:31

W e will start by defining the end goal, and then we will work backward to build the plan. From this point forward, your goal when eating, for the rest of your life, is this:

I will eat a diet made primarily of foods as God created them. This diet will be as low in added sugar as possible and without processed ingredients or chemicals (including MSG). It will be low in total carbohydrates and gluten free. The majority of my nutrition will come from healthy fats, natural meats, colorful vegetables, and fruit. I will eat based on the rule that what I put into my body either makes me more healthy or less healthy. I will maximize nutrition and minimize toxicity.

Before we get too far into the details, we need to talk about tracking your food intake. I mentioned earlier using the app MyFitnessPal (or MyNetDiary). This is an easy way to track what you eat. You need to do this for at least one week before starting this plan, to set a baseline. You should then track your intake throughout the seven weeks as directed in the worksheets, which are included in Part II. The app should also be used periodically after completing the seven weeks of the plan to help you stay accountable and on track.

As I mentioned earlier, the most important details we will track are total carbohydrates, added sugar, and the percentage of your calories that come from fats, carbohydrates, and protein in your diet. Goals for each of these are listed later. Please become accustomed to using this app (or another way of tracking your dietary intake).

This way of eating will lead to dramatic internal and external improvements in your health. I am excited for you. You are worth the effort you are about to put into restoring your temple. Now how will you get there? Let's find out.

There are ten rules that apply from day one and that we will build upon. Remember this will not seem easy at first. Don't give in—no cheating yourself on any of these. Once you see and feel the changes, this will prove to be one of the best decisions you have ever made. But before we get to the rules, let me remind you of a few things and let you in on a disclaimer.

First, this is not a *diet* in the sense that the word diet relates to a short-term weight-loss plan or fad. I use the word diet as defined by Merriam-Webster: "food and drink regularly provided or consumed." This is the way humans should sustain themselves, based on eating foods as God created them. Unfortunately, this is not how the majority of Americans currently eat. If you want to continue to eat like everyone else, you can expect to experience what they do. It is possible our children are the first generation that will be less healthy and have a shorter life span than their parents.

It is often said that the definition of *insanity* is doing the same thing over and over while expecting different results. This is your opportunity to do something different so you can expect different results.

Over two-thirds of Americans are overweight or obese. The number of adults with type 2 diabetes is out of control. This was once known as adult-onset diabetes because until about twenty years ago zero children were diagnosed with this diet-related disease. Now over fifty thousand American children are diabetic because of the foods we are feeding them.[1] Cancer rates are on the rise. Alzheimer's rates are rising (and it is being diagnosed at a younger average age). In a sad summary, many chronic, debilitating adult and pediatric diseases are becoming more prevalent. This all correlates with major changes in what we eat and how processed the "foods" we eat are.

The Standard American Diet has the initials SAD. It is sad. The overall health of our society is in a sad state. It is declining precipitously. This Restore Your Temple diet, based on foods God has created, as He created them, is your chance to restore your health. It will deliver the positive results you need.

An interesting thing however happens when you live differently. People begin to question and challenge the choices you make. They feel uncomfortable, and they want to say you are wrong so they don't have to be introspective. They don't feel the need to have their own evidence when they challenge you for yours. This holds true if you are eating differently, loving your family differently, or following Christ.

I believe God made it this way for a reason. It gives us the opportunity to speak truth into other people's lives when they see us living differently and question us on it.

First, people will ask for your proof. Almost always, however, they do not have proof themselves for the choices *they* are making. Remember that eating the way everyone else eats is also a choice. We all know (if we take the time to think about it) what the outcome of that decision is. Almost 10 percent of American adults are diabetic, and the number is growing each year.[2] In addition to diabetes, Cancer, Alzheimer's, depression, autoimmune diseases, and many other diseases have gone from nearly nonexistent 100 years ago to extremely prevalent. It seems fair to ask why?

Diabetes

Diabetes is increasing in the US, but a healthy lifestyle can often prevent or delay the onset of diabetes.

USA Diabetes (1996-2014) see more

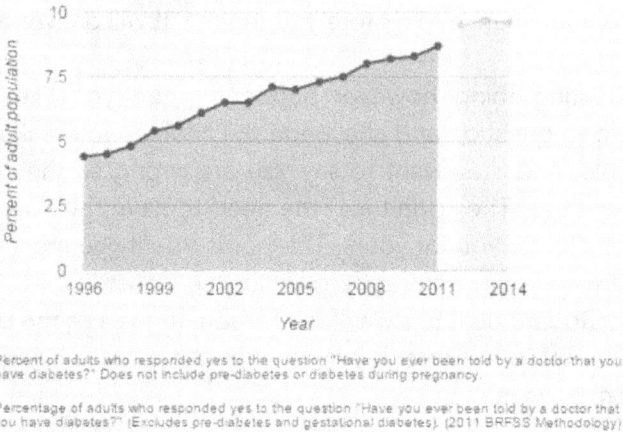

Percent of adults who responded yes to the question "Have you ever been told by a doctor that you have diabetes?" Does not include pre-diabetes or diabetes during pregnancy.

Percentage of adults who responded yes to the question "Have you ever been told by a doctor that you have diabetes?" (Excludes pre-diabetes and gestational diabetes). (2011 BRFSS Methodology)

Think about this: when the American diet is "exported" and becomes the new way of eating in other cultures, the outcome is disastrous. "No country in the world has the resources to continue to treat diabetics the way that they're being treated now, if the prevalence rates increase at the rates that they're increasing for much longer," says physician and author Kevin Patterson.[3] We just don't see it as readily ourselves here in America because we are living in the middle of it. So my response is this: I see the proof of what will happen if we continue to eat like everyone else, and I want nothing to do with it for me or my family.

Second, people will present "facts" and challenge you to answer to them. They are going to question whether these healthy fats should be a major part of your diet. For example, "You are going to get fat if you eat too many fatty foods." Not true if they are the right fatty foods. Or "Your cholesterol is going to be a problem if you eat this way." Myth. In fact, the opposite may actually be true. The list is endless.

Look at what happened to obesity rates in America about the time we started recommending a "low-fat" diet.[4]

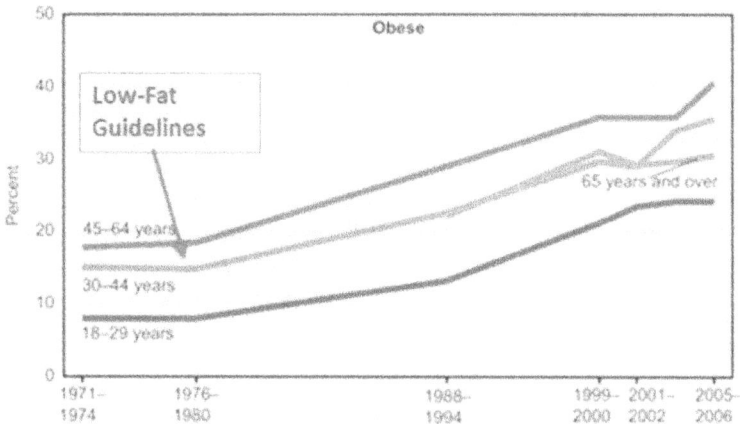

The food industry has turned food into nothing more than a commodity. They took something God created for our good and made it into something we desire for the wrong reasons. They made it into a money maker. We now desire food because of the sugar, gluten, and chemicals in it. Not because we are actually hungry or because of the way it nourishes our bodies. Isn't it interesting that obese people seem to always be hungry? Does that make any sense? These foods in many ways are like illicit drugs. We need to think this way, especially when we feed them to our families.

Here is my disclaimer: I have taken ideas from many places and co-alesced them into this life-changing restoration plan. I truly believe this will work for you in dramatic and measurable ways. If there is a plan or research available, I have likely read it. There is so much information out there, and I know that can be overwhelming. If you would like to do the more detailed research on your own, here are just a few of my resources:

- Bible
- Makers Diet
- Rice Diet
- Bulletproof Diet

- Whole 30 Plan
- Paleo Diet
- Grain Brain
- Wheat Belly
- *Fed Up* (movie)
- Adrenal Reset Diet
- Medical literature reviews
- Many more

I will leave the details and reasoning for these to the respective sources, which you can read. Here, I hope to simplify the somewhat overwhelming information for you so you can quickly implement changes to your life.

So here are the rules you must learn, understand, and incorporate into your life. Each has sound research backing, details of which can be found in the recommended resources. Note that to make following these rules easier, a full shopping list is also provided in the appendix.

There is one more thing I should mention before we get to the rules. I am not saying that eating any other way is a sin. This is a plan for optimizing your health by eating foods as God created them. It is not necessarily a salvation issue. Everything God created is good, if used as He intended it to be used and in a way that glorifies Him. Many of the foods available to us, however, are processed or diminished versions of His creation. I hope this plan helps you to eat in a way that restores your health. I am confident it will.

The Rules

1. Limit added sugars in your diet to near elimination.

Sugar is added to nearly everything in our current diet. Food companies started doing this over the last twenty years, and I believe this is one of the primary reasons for many health issues in our culture. At the very least, sugar consumption increases your risk of obesity, diabetes, and heart disease.

Interestingly, Connecticut College Professor Joseph Schroeder performed a study comparing Oreos to cocaine or morphine. He and his students found rats formed as strong an association with the effects of eating Oreos and as they did cocaine or morphine. They also found that eating the sugar- (and wheat-) filled cookies activated more neurons in the brain's pleasure center than exposure to drugs of abuse. Schroeder said, "It may explain why some people can't resist these foods despite the fact that they know they are bad for them." It is also telling that the rats ate the Oreos in the same way many humans do—they opened the Oreo and ate the middle first.[5]

No wonder the industry has created multiple names for sugar in ingredient lists! To help you remove them from your diet, I've listed them in the appendix. Whatever the name, total added sugar should be less than thirty grams a day and as close to zero as possible. Each food you eat should have less than five grams of added sugar per serving. This can be tracked on MyFitnessPal or by reading food labels. There is an exception: you should have three servings of actual God-created fruit per day, and these sugars do not count toward the total of less than thirty grams per day.

One caution: do not replace the sugar with sugar-free or diet alternatives. Those are also off limits. Absolutely no aspartame (NutraSweet), sucralose (Splenda), or acesulfame potassium. Xylitol from American hardwoods is an alternative to sugar that can be used in the occasional recipe.

2. Remove MSG and other chemically altered ingredients from your diet.

This includes monosodium glutamate (MSG) by all of its names. Food manufacturers have found ways to manufacture MSG by other names in order to get it into your food. It should be completely eliminated. I have included a list in the appendix of all of the different types of free glutamate that are added to foods. Take it with you shopping. Use it to clean out your pantry and refrigerator. If these ingredients are in your food, do not eat it.

Also limit sulfites and nitrites.

3. Remove gluten from your diet.

This includes wheat flour, rye, barley, and bran, which should be completely eliminated.

You might ask, "Isn't wheat natural?" Dr. William Davis, author of *Wheat Belly*, has this to say about the current "wheat" used in our diets.

> First of all, it ain't wheat. It's the product of 40 years of genetics research aimed at increasing yield-per-acre. The result is a genetically unique plant that stands 18–24 inches tall, not the 4 1/2-foot tall 'amber waves of grain' we all remember. The genetic distance modern wheat has drifted exceeds the difference between chimpanzees and humans.[6]

This genetically altered version of wheat that we now consume—some call it Frankenwheat—has up to three times the gluten, which potentially leads to inflammation, many auto-immune diseases, and thyroid disorders like Hashimoto's Disease. It also contains a starch called amylopectin, which the body has trouble converting into energy. It therefore stores it as fat. This is likely a major contributor to the diabetes, Alzheimer's disease, and obesity epidemics we now face as a nation.

Wheat, like sugar, is also addictive. It makes you want to eat more and crave more. This is unfortunate, since there is strong or growing evidence that the following are possibly symptoms or issues associated with gluten sensitivity:

- ADHD
- Anxiety
- Ataxia
- Autism
- Autoimmune disorders including Hashimoto's thyroiditis and multiple types of arthritis
- Osteoporosis
- Brain fog
- Multiple cancers
- Depression

- Bowel and digestive issues
- Bloating and gas
- Constipation
- Irritable Bowel Syndrome
- Migraine and other headaches
- History of miscarriage
- Multiple neurologic disorders such as Alzheimer's and other forms of dementia, schizophrenia, and Parkinsonism
- Seizures

Other carbohydrates like oats (gluten-free only), rice, buckwheat, quinoa, coconut flour, and other gluten-free flours can be eaten on a limited basis. However, do not assume replacing gluten with packaged, gluten-free alternatives is always a healthy decision. Many of those options are not healthy and do not fit into the rules of your new way of eating.

Your optimal total carbohydrates should be less than one hundred grams. However a good goal is one hundred to one hundred fifty grams.

4. Limit dairy.

This includes cow's milk, cream, cream cheese, yogurt, and sour cream, which should be used sparingly and in grass-fed, organic, and full-fat forms when at all possible. Do not substitute in light or skim versions.

An exception is cultured organic butter and ghee. These can and should be used often. They are included in the healthy fats that will be a major part of your diet. Grass-fed butter is a great option for making food taste awesome.

5. Limit your ingredients.

Most of your diet should consist of one-ingredient foods from the included shopping list. There are few exceptions to this, in which case you should try to limit ingredients of food purchases to no more than three ingredients. For example, if purchasing black beans, the ingredients may be black beans, water, and salt.

Of course, none of the ingredients should be added sugar—at least not above five grams per serving—or the chemically modified ingredients discussed above.

You should have heard of the ingredients in the foods you are eating. This is best accomplished by spending the majority of your shopping time in the outer part of the grocery store where whole foods are commonly found, not the aisles filled with processed foods.

6. Limit your alcohol.

You should not consume any alcohol for the first three weeks. Here is a good place to exhibit your willpower. Learn to say no and to live with no excuses.

After the first three weeks the goal will be as follows:

- Optimal amount is zero to two drinks per week
- Maximum amount is three to four drinks per week

A drink is a twelve-ounce beer (gluten free), a five-ounce serving of wine, or 1.5 ounces of distilled spirits. Make sure your alcohol use is in responsible, God-honoring environments and situations.

7. Do not count calories.

All calories are not the same! So I do not care about total calories. One hundred calories of coconut oil is so different from one hundred calories of sugar that it is not even worth comparing them. However, your percent of calories that come from fat, protein, and carbohydrates is important. The optimal dietary calorie intake in percentage form is as follows:

- 50–70 percent of calories from healthy fats
- 20–30 percent of calories from protein
- Less than 30 percent of calories from carbohydrates

8. Eat lots of healthy fat and organic or grass-fed proteins (meat and eggs).

Get over the myth that eating fats will make you fat. Seriously, get over it. These will be the majority of your diet, along with vegetables. These healthy fats and proteins are listed in the included shopping list.

9. Eat lots of vegetables.

This is very important: you should be consuming seven to ten servings per day. As far as defining what is a fruit or a vegetable, go with the list that is provided later. Just make sure it's fresh or frozen, not canned. I also have included a list (in the appendix) of the fruits and vegetables that you should be purchasing in their organic form.

10. Eat three servings of God-created fruits in their God-created forms.

This means no fruit juice. None! Eat the fruit in the form God made it. Use the provided list.

So there it is. Now that you have the details and approved shopping list (in the appendix), I will simplify the steps you will take.

- Clean out your cabinets and refrigerator of anything that does not follow the rules or anything that is not on the shopping list (demolition week).
- Use the shopping list to determine and plan what you will eat.
- Shop following the ten rules and using the shopping list.
- Experiment and learn to eat the way you are supposed to.
- Completely transform your health and body.
- Don't turn back.

This is a big step for you, I am sure. It is scary because it is different, and there are unknowns. You're wondering how you are going to eat and what you are going to eat. Here is my encouragement to you: *It is worth it! You are worth it! Your health is worth it! Restore your temple!*

Also, if it helps, in the appendix I have included an example day in my life as far as my diet goes to give you an idea of how I eat. I would also like to note that I currently drink Bulletproof Coffee[7] in the mornings, as my breakfast. As I said, my diet is a conglomeration of components of many diets and the Bulletproof Diet is one of them. For simplicity sake, my version of Bulletproof Coffee is ten ounces of coffee (brewed with an Aeropress) made with freshly ground USDA organic beans. This is then blended with one tablespoon of ghee (or grass-fed butter), one table-spoon of Bulletproof Brain Octane Oil (or coconut oil), and sometimes one teaspoon of organic pure cacao powder. It is my breakfast (along with vitamin D and R--Alpha Lipoic acid). This amounts to about three hundred calories of healthy fat, vitamins, very little sugar, and some caffeine. This may be something you consider, especially if you are a coffee drinker.

Another topic we should discuss is fasting. I suggest you research this on your own. There are many benefits to fasting, and it is a biblically sound practice. An occasional fast will give you insight into how food and other things in your life control you. We are to be sustained by the Word, not food.

Biblically, there are fasts lasting from one day to forty days. You could start with a partial fast from breakfast to breakfast. In this type of fast, you skip lunch and dinner.

Finally, if necessary in specific situations (traveling, parties, or when feeding your kids/other family members), you can consider using a 10 per-cent rule. This means that at a birthday party or when traveling you look at it this way: give yourself 10 percent leeway if needed to keep yourself on track. It would be best, of course, to not do this if at all possible. It also does not mean that 10 percent of the foods in your home or on a normal day should be outside of the rules. This applies to special situations only.

There are actually a few benefits to this idea.

- It will allow you to feel less "crazy" when trying to eat right in our culture. This small amount of leeway can provide some grace to you in these specific situations.
- You will experience what the foods you are now avoiding with the restoration eating plan have been doing to your body for many years. After eating by the restoration plan for a while you will feel

better and begin to crave health-promoting food. You will literally become less toxic. Your body will like being nourished the way it is meant to be. You will also become less tolerant to the toxins you were previously eating because your body will now "know better." This experience will further reinforce eating the right way. The subtle brain fog, stomach ache, headache, or just not feeling right will become noticeable, instead of normal.

This is the diet that will restore your body as a temple. If early on you cannot find much to eat, it is still better than eating the processed chemicals that are now called "food." Hunger is relative and is mind-over-matter in many ways. After removing many addictive and artificial ingredients from your diet and adding healthy fats, your experience with hunger will likely change. You will grow in confidence by overcoming this for you and your family.

I challenge you to take an all-in approach to this. Your success will be greatly determined by your initial decision to commit, your support system (more on this later), and the results I know you will experience.

BUILDING BLOCK 3

Exercise: Strengthen Your Temple

*For physical training is of some value, but godliness
has value for all things, holding promise for
both the present life and the life to come.*
1 TIMOTHY *4:8*

E xercise is an important part of restoring your temple, but needs to be kept in context. We live in a sedentary culture and many of us sit or do little physical activity during our day. Therefore setting time aside for dedicated physical activity is good and, for many, necessary. This needs to be part of a plan in which we are also training for godliness, as Paul says in his letter to Timothy. This restoration plan will be exactly that for you.

Exercise will help you return your body to health in many ways. Of course, physical fitness and, for some, weight loss are desirable outcomes of exercise. Exercise also has secondary benefits such as improving mood, awareness, confidence, time management, and energy levels. It can also decrease the risk of heart attack and osteoporosis.

Like the other building blocks, exercise alone will not produce lasting or meaningful change. Complete restoration for you will mean implementing all seven building blocks and building them upon the cornerstone of your life: Christ. That being said, here is how we will implement this building block into your life over the next seven weeks.

You will exercise thirty minutes per day at least three days per week. Note the minimal number of days for exercise is three per week; for additional benefit you may choose up to six.

Your exercise plan will be split into three categories: strength, stamina, and flexibility/body-weight training. The most important of these for overall benefit is the strength category and should be implemented right away. This is especially true for those of you who exercise the minimal number of days per week.

Let's look at each category separately.

Strength training is extremely important for overall health no matter your age or gender. This does not mean you are training to become a bodybuilder or to gain huge muscle mass. However, adding muscle to your temple has many benefits. Having muscle increases your metabolism, helps you maintain a healthy bone structure and composition, and will help you maintain a healthy weight. Also, being stronger is just plain fun.

Stamina training (or cardiovascular exercise) is also an important part of a training routine. It should, however, not take the place of strength training or be done in excess. Cardiovascular training will increase your overall health. It also makes it easier for you to perform tasks of daily living or other things you enjoy.

Flexibility (or body-weight training) is a broad category of training that can be performed separately or as part of the other two categories. Maintaining flexibility will help you limit injuries and perform movement-based activities. When paired with body-weight training, you will build a strong core, which has many additional benefits.

How will these three training methods look in your restoration plan as you implement exercise into your life? Just like the rest of the building blocks, success in this area starts with having a plan, as well as short-term and long-term goals. Then you will need to have the willpower to make exercise a prioritized part of your life.

The plan will be incorporated into the weekly worksheets for the next seven weeks. No excuses. You need to put at least three thirty-minute blocks into your schedule to be used solely for exercise. I recommend five or six for optimal results. Get ready to change your body and your attitude. Again, this restoration project is physical, emotional, and spiritual.

I don't feel like I need to reinvent the wheel as far as setting up a unique Restore Your Temple exercise program. There are many commercially available options for home video-based training. You could also join a gym or follow your own plan. But for the sake of completeness, and potentially to guide some of you who need it, I will give you a brief outline of what I do. If you want to go ahead and copy my plan, I have put time into developing it and think it would be an efficient plan for you to use.

In short, my time for dedicated exercise is six-thirty a.m. (after my time of prayer in the morning) on weekdays and sometimes Saturday. I primarily use Beachbody videos and have come up with my own routine that combines a few of their video series to best implement the fundamentals previously outlined. (I should mention here that I am not currently a Beachbody coach or affiliated with them.) The series I currently use are P90X3 and PiYo (and sometimes P90X). P90X3 is primarily used for strength and stamina training. PiYo is used for primarily flexibility and body-weight training.

I feel like I should briefly talk about yoga, since the PiYo video series is loosely based on yoga training. As a follower of Jesus, I understand the objection some Christians have against yoga as a form of exercise. I wholeheartedly agree that yoga as a lifestyle modification program, with all of its religious and spiritual implications, should not be used by followers of Jesus. However, I feel that is not the focus of the PiYo video series, and I therefore don't feel like there is issue with using this specific series solely for exercise purposes.

So what does my plan look like? I have included my weekly plan in the appendix. I have also included a generic exercise plan. You can use either of these as your plan or the backbone for making your own plan. The key, however, is to dedicate yourself to working for thirty minutes at least three times per week.

There are innumerable benefits to incorporating exercise into your life. The key to obtaining these benefits can be summed up by the Nike slogan, "Just Do It." Interestingly, one of the secondary benefits to exercise is stress reduction, which is our next building block.

BUILDING BLOCK 4

Stress Reduction: Find Peace for Your Soul

The Lord is my shepherd, I lack nothing.
He makes me lie down in green pastures,
he leads me beside quiet waters,
he refreshes my soul.
He guides me along the right paths
for his name's sake.
Even though I walk
through the darkest valley,
I will fear no evil,
for you are with me;
your rod and your staff,
they comfort me.
PSALM 23:1-4

Wow. We live in a stressed-out culture. David's words from Psalm 23 are reason to believe it does not have to be this way. We don't need to live under the constant strain and emotional struggle that many of us do. So how do we find peace for our soul and rest for our mind? That is exactly what you will find out in this part of the restoration plan.

The American Psychological Society published the results[8] from their "Stress in America" report and let's just say Americans need some peace. Here are a few of the highlights (or lowlights):

- The majority of Americans report experiencing some symptoms of stress—67 percent report experiencing emotional symptoms of stress and 72 percent report experiencing physical symptoms of stress.
- 61 percent of adults say managing stress is extremely or very important, but only 35 percent say they are doing an excellent or very good job at it.
- 27 percent of adults say they eat to manage stress, and 34 percent of those who report overeating or eating unhealthy foods because of stress say this behavior is a habit.
- 43 percent of American adults report stress has caused them to lie awake at night in the past month alone.

So why are Americans so discontent? What is going on that we, as a culture, are so unhappy? How can you overcome this?

I truly believe you have found the answer by committing yourself to restoration of your mind, body, and soul. The Lord is good, and He loves you. As David discovered in his previously quoted psalm, when we are focused on the Lord, the cares of this world diminish. When we walk on the path He has made clear for us, we will not be distressed by the troubles of this life. It is all about our focus. When we focus on the world, we are engulfed by the stress of the world. When we focus on the Lord, we are surrounded by His grace.

Read the following biblical truths and tell me one good reason not to believe me on this matter:

- *"Cast all your anxiety on him because he cares for you"* (1 Peter 5:7).
- *"Come to me, all you who are weary and burdened, and I will give you rest"* (Matthew 11:28).
- *"Do not conform to the pattern of this world, but be transformed by the renewing of your mind. Then you will be able to test and approve what God's will is—his good, pleasing and perfect will"* (Romans 12:2).
- *"Peace I leave with you; my peace I give you. I do not give to you as the world gives. Do not let your hearts be troubled and do not be afraid"* (John 14:27).

Read and re-read those. Memorize them. Save them on your Bible app. The world would like to tell you to handle stress yourself or overcome stress with the help of other people or medications. I ask you, what does the God who created you say you should do with your stress?

I have one more for you to read. I think it really hammers the point home:

> *Do not be anxious about anything, but in every situation, by prayer and petition, with thanksgiving, present your requests to God. And the peace of God, which transcends all understanding, will guard your hearts and your minds in Christ Jesus.* (Philippians 4:6–7)

Are you ready to get there? This building block is a bit different from the others. This part of the plan will not rely on your own effort. Instead, you will be learning to let some things go, to loosen your grip. God is in control and has you in His hands. He wants you to know Him. He wants you to rely on Him. He wants you to know and obey His word. That is where true peace is found. It is also where health can be restored: *"A heart at peace gives life to the body, but envy rots the bones"* (Proverbs 14:30).

Let's take a look at the steps you will be taking over the next seven weeks to move you into a closer relationship with the One who can take your burdens.

Prayer Journal

As part of building block number one, you will already be praying and making prayer a substantial part of your daily life. This prayer will take place during dedicated time in the morning, to start your day. At night, you will be journaling about the workings of the Lord in your life and through your prayers. This will be an exercise in awareness. It will also help you put into words the many ways God is restoring you to the extraordinary person He created you to be. Finally, it will serve as a reminder in regard to the growth you are making, as you will be able to look back upon your journal entries and reflect.

Each night you will journal on the following three things:

- List three things you are thankful for today.
- In what way did you best restore your temple today?
- How did you see God work in your life today?

Music

I cannot emphasize enough how much music has calmed my soul and guided my heart. The music you listen to, TV/movies you watch, and Web sites/social media you visit set the tone for your day. They guide your attitude and thoughts for the day. You may not think that those things alter who you are, but they most definitely do. So what would happen if the soundtrack of your life became words of hope, love, and salvation? What if you were singing along to songs that worship your Savior instead of music telling you to worship yourself or some other person or thing? I can tell you that for me, it has been life changing.

For the next seven weeks we are going to try this together. I will guide you further on this in the weekly worksheets, but for now, if your local area has a Christian radio station, set it up in your vehicle. If you listen to music in your home, use that opportunity to worship the One who cared enough to give His life for you. No matter if on Pandora, the radio, iTunes, or wherever you listen to music, for the next seven weeks let your ears and mind be filled with the peace of the Lord. I will also recommend two songs for each week in the worksheets.

Perspective

Stress and worry are a matter of perspective. Let me give you a practical example of this. On a recent December afternoon, I was walking out of church and it was about 50 degrees outside. It was sort of damp, and there was a light fog. This was unseasonably warm for a mid-December day in Wisconsin. People were giddy. No coats or hats. They were making plans to be out in the yard and spending time outside. So from the perspective that it was supposed to be very cold and dry, people were happy about this 50-degree foggy and damp day.

Now, what if it was mid-July and those same people were planning an outdoor wedding? Would they be giddy and excited about 50 degrees, fog, and potential rain? I expect not. I would imagine there would be some worry and complaining.

Stress is a matter of perspective. When your perspective is the reality that God is in control, He loves you, and He will carry your burdens, it changes everything. Let me repeat that: God is in control. He loves you. He will carry your burdens, and you can cast your anxiety on Him: *"Now may the Lord of peace himself give you peace at all times and in every way. The Lord be with all of you"* (2 Thessalonians 3:16).

What are you worried about again?

My hope is that you can experience this profound truth. I can barely put into words how different my life is now that I understand it. This world cannot give us peace and happiness; without Him it is impossible. All other peace and happiness is temporary or misplaced; He is never ending. Think about that. He loves you and always will, always and forever. What is there to be worried about if we really believe this?

Understanding this changes everything. It even makes our relationships (with our spouse, kids, and Christian friends) much better. Oh, how it has changed my marriage and my parenting to have this peace. I also am a much better friend now. This understanding helps me to define what a true friend is. It puts others needs into perspective. We are called to love others. How can anyone do that if they do not know the love of the Father? I pray that we all can experience Him and His peace to the utmost.

Another way to help you to live a life with less stress and more reliance on the God who loves you is to surround yourself with people who will support you and build you up. This brings us to the next chapter.

BUILDING BLOCK 5

Community: Choose Your Companions

And let us consider how we may spur one another on toward love and good deeds, not giving up meeting together, as some are in the habit of doing, but encouraging one another—and all the more as you see the Day approaching.
HEBREWS 10:24–25

M uch of the Restore Your Temple plan is about restoring yourself and your relationship with God. This is extremely important and a good place to start. Jesus, however, was asked what the greatest commandment was. He replied,

> *"Love the Lord your God with all your heart and with all your soul and with all your mind." This is the first and greatest commandment. And the second is like it: "Love your neighbor as yourself." All the Law and the Prophets hang on these two commandments.* (Matthew 22:37–40)

As you see, the second part of that involves our relationships with others. We spend most of our time with others. Those relationships shape us and can allow us opportunity. As part of your restoration plan, we will take a look at how these relationships can lead you (and hopefully others) further down the path the Lord has paved for you.

Hierarchy of Relationships

The Bible gives us principles that allow us to order our relationships in a healthy manner. Each relationship we have is of importance. However, some are to be held in higher regard than others. More time and effort need to go into certain relationships than into others. If we get this order out of balance, our temple will crumble. Our relationships will suffer. So what does this hierarchy look like?

God

As Jesus stated in the previous scripture, our relationship with the Lord is first and foremost. Ignoring this fact will lead to serious consequences and is the etiology of most of the ills of our culture. This restoration plan will help you to place your relationship with God in the proper place—at the top of your priority list. This should be evident in the way you spend your time, talents, and resources.

Spouse

The next most important relationship, if you are married, is with your spouse. A married man is to love his wife as Christ loved the church (see Ephesians 5:25). Christ loved the Father with his utmost. His second priority was His church. Men are to love their wives in the same manner. Wives are to submit to their husbands "as you do to the Lord" (Ephesians 5:22). Therefore a woman's husband is second only to God in her priorities.

Children

A husband and wife are one flesh (see Ephesians 5:31) and children are often the result of marriage; your children are therefore the next priority.

As parents, we are called to raise godly children who love the Lord their God with all their hearts (see Ephesians 6:4).

Parents

The Bible is also very clear with the command we are to love and honor our parents. Therefore our parents (no matter their age) are to come next.

Extended Family/Fellow Believers

Our extended families fall in line at this point, followed by other fellow believers.

The Rest

Finally comes the rest of the people in the world (see Matt 28:19), with whom we should be focused on bringing the gospel and making disciples of Christ. Of note, if family members are not followers of Christ they also fit into this last category.

So in summary our relationships should be structured as such:

1. God
2. Spouse (if married)
3. Your children
4. Parents
5. Extended family
6. Fellow Christians
7. Non-Christians

Those higher on the list should get more of your time, care, and attention. If a relationship is breaking down or suffering, the effort on that relationship should be the priority and not those below it on the list. Oh, the troubles our culture could prevent if only by following this simple truth!

Relational Circles

You can also think of this concept as relational circles. The circles in the center are those relationships of highest priority. They are the closest relationships to you. They are also the ones most influential and stabilizing in the maintenance of your temple. The further away from the center a relationship is the less of your time and attention it should get. Those relationships further away from the center should also have less access to the personal and intimate details of your life. Your needs, desires, and counsel should be reserved for only your "inner circles."

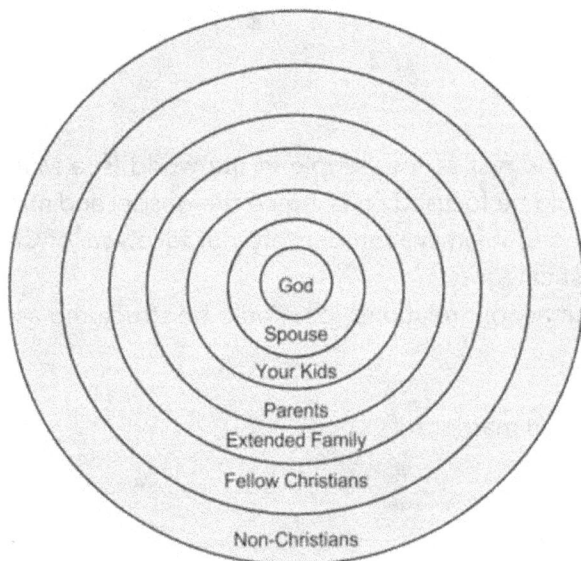

Bible Study Groups

Another awesome way to build community and grow in your relationship with the Lord is through a Bible-based small group. Meeting regularly with other believers is a fundamental Christian principle that has been greatly diminished in our society. The benefits of this are endless. It promotes growth with accountability. It strengthens your knowledge of the Word.

It builds a sense of family with other Christians, which pays off in times of need or celebration. This can be done with other couples and/or in men's/ women's small group settings. I cannot understate how much I believe in the need for small group gathering with other Christians. Maybe the most important benefit of these times is that God tells us He is present when we gather in this way: *"For where two or three gather in my name, there am I with them"* (Matthew 18:20).

Social Media

How does social media fit into this? Let's start with the recent statistic from The Buntin Group, which found the average time Americans spend per week on social media is twenty-three hours.[9] That's about 14 percent of the week. Much of that time is given to those in our outer circles. Imagine if we took that time and devoted it to interactions with God, our spouses, and those we love.

In our culture, we are constantly inundated by media. The Internet is everywhere and our minds are being filled with ideas and imagery through multiple sources. As mentioned previously, the average American is spending a significant proportion of their week being "entertained" by the media. Eventually, these constant distractions and overload of information change us. They affect us in ways we do not even realize.

Step one is just being aware of it. Then step two is purposeful usage or limitation. We need to curtail how much of our time we give to social media, television, and other forms of "entertainment." We need to be present in our relationships. For the purposes of our temple restoration plan, we will not spend more time on our phones, computers, or televisions than we are spending doing one of the following three things:

- Time in prayer or study (Building Block 1)
- Time exercising (Building Block 3)
- Time in community with those at the top of our hierarchy list (Building Block 5)

Does this make sense? The total amount of time in a day you spend on your electronics needs to be less than the time spent on these three temple building blocks. This is a minimum goal. Obviously the more time spent on the building blocks, the better. This is the challenge for this building block.

I would like to conclude this section about the building block of community with a quote from Life Church pastor Craig Groeschel. He said, "Show me your friends, and I will show you your future." I truly believe this can be expanded into the entirety of our relationships. Make sure you have your priorities in order in regard to your relationships. You are going to need help restoring and maintaining your temple. The people with whom you choose to embark on this adventure will greatly influence the outcome of your restoration.

BUILDING BLOCK 6

Removing Toxins:
Cleanse Your Life

We have already discussed at length how we will change what we are putting into our bodies through our mouths. By following the diet building block, the number of toxins entering your body will be greatly diminished. There are other ways toxins enter our bodies, however. We will be discussing a few of those here and what steps you will take to eliminate these toxins.

Smoking

The first and most obvious toxin I want to discuss is tobacco. This one will be easy for me because there is no question or debate as to the action you need to take on this. If you are smoking (or chewing) tobacco, you need to stop. There are many different programs, patches, and devices out there to assist you in this. No matter which you use, it will also require a support system (Building Block 5) and some intense prayer (Building Block 1). This section is short because this is so obvious. Your life will be similarly short if you continue to use this toxin. Let me say it one more time: you need to stop. Forever.

Cleaning Supplies

Our cleaning supplies are fraught with danger. Many chemicals you use around the house are made of things you would never allow to be in your home if you knew what they were. The workers who make the supplies in some cases have to be protected while handling them before they ship them out for you to spray all around your home. This is something I could go on and on about. Here is my advice to you: start thinking about these products and use the Environmental Working Group website (www.ewg.org) to search the products you currently own and ones you are considering. Then replace them with less toxic options.

Deodorant and Cosmetics

I have similar things to say about cosmetics. However, this one may be more urgent since you apply these directly to your body. Again, I would encourage you to research this a bit on your own and use www.ewg.org.

I would also recommend watching the video *Story of Cosmetics*. Search the Internet for it. There is some debate about the use of antiperspirants and their effect on your health. Nevertheless, this is something most of us use every day, so choosing a more natural deodorant cannot hurt. This is where I recommend you start this challenge.

Aromatherapy

- *"Is anyone among you sick? Let them call the elders of the church to pray over them and anoint them with oil in the name of the Lord"* (James 5:14).
- *"Fruit trees of all kinds will grow on both banks of the river. Their leaves will not wither, nor will their fruit fail. Every month they will bear fruit, because the water from the sanctuary flows to them. Their fruit will serve for food and their leaves for healing"* (Ezekiel 47:12).

Essential oils and herbs were often used and referenced in the Bible. If you are interested in replacing some of the toxins in your home with a more natural and beneficial alternative, natural oils and scents are great options. They can take the place of some of the artificial smells in our lotions, candles, and perfumes. They can also be used for relaxation and healing. I will not go into great detail here and recommend you do some research on this topic if interested. I will however provide the following in the appendix.

- A list of supplies to give you a kick start into the use of essential oils.
- A few recipes for:
  - a relaxation inhaler
  - a room spray
  - a hand sanitizer
- I also recommend using an ionic essential oil diffuser in your home.

Removing obvious and hidden toxins in your life can provide great health benefit. Many of these toxins lead to chronic low-level irritation, symptoms, and in some cases even disease. You may not see immediate, obvious benefit; however, the benefits provided are an important part of your overall restoration plan.

BUILDING BLOCK 7

Rest and Worship: Reset Your Compass

> *By the seventh day God had finished the work he had been doing; so on the seventh day he rested from all his work.*
> GENESIS 2:2

Rest is an extremely important part of this restoration project you are undertaking. Rest comes in many forms: physical, emotional, mental, and soulful. We will carefully consider all of these and how to incorporate them into your life, as well as some of the benefits of doing so.

Sleep

The most obvious form of rest is sleep. C.S. Lewis once said, "You don't have a soul. You are a soul. You have a body." Unfortunately sometimes our bodies become a limitation. They get tired and worn down. They need rest.

We will incorporate rest and sleep into your life, but we will also tackle your lack of restfulness from another angle. This plan will revitalize your soul. It will add health and stamina to your body. This means you will likely feel less tired and your need for sleep may change. You will have to determine what an appropriate and healthy amount of sleep is for you and then make sure you are getting it. In addition, there are apps to help with that. I recommend the smartphone app called Sleep Cycle or the sleep tracking element of a fitness tracking band if you want to monitor your sleep more closely.

Rest for your Body

Sunday should be a day of bodily rest for you. We will not exercise on Sunday and, if at all possible, you should try to limit the amount you work on Sundays. If not Sunday, then choose another day of the week that works for you. You need a day to recuperate. If God felt he needed to rest one day a week, it seems fitting that we should do the same.

Worship

A very important component of rest is spiritual rejuvenation. Your soul needs to be refreshed. Your compass needs to be reset. Your attitude needs to be readjusted. Your path needs to be made clear. These things can best be accomplished through the worship of our Lord and Savior. I cannot underestimate the importance of worship. It is the act of showing reverence, adoration, and admiration to God. If you truly believe in your heart He is God, and you trust Him with your life, worship will surely follow. You will worship because your soul desires it. You will worship because He deserves your praise. You will worship in preparation for eternity with Him. You will worship because you will be overcome with joy and amazement at the gift He has given you.

My challenge to you is this: if you are not worshiping the Lord on a regular basis, do you really believe in Him? Do you really trust Him? Do you know Him? If you did, worship would be obvious to you. You would feel the desire and need to worship Him.

My challenge to you is to find a place to worship the Lord with other believers. Notice I did not say go to church. Just "going to church" can be a ritualistic activity. However, finding a church where you can worship the Lord with other believers is life changing. You can only know that if you experience it. Once you experience it you will desire the opportunity to show Him on a regular basis how much you love Him. Find a place where you can do that and do so at least three to four times per month. This may be a challenge for you initially but will soon become your soul's desire.

If you need help finding a church, ask around. Find a believer you relate with and find out where he or she goes to church. Do not feel bad trying out a few different churches. Ask yourself some questions about a church to see if it is a fit for you. The one thing I would like to stress however is this: God will let you know. You will feel it in your heart and soul if you are in the right place. When you find a place to truly worship Him, it will feel right.

Here are four questions to help:

- Is this a church where I feel I am being taught God's Word?
- Is this a church where I can worship and feel the presence of God?
- Is this a church where my family will experience meaningful Christian fellowship and accountability?
- Is this a church where I will have the opportunity to serve God's people and use my gifts for His benefit?

Charity

One very powerful way to restore your temple and rest your soul is to give. Give of your time, talent, and finances. Give, most important, to *"the least of these"* (Matthew 25:40). Those who are in need—the orphans, widows, and sick, the poor and hungry. In a radical and awesome statement on the importance of giving of oneself Jesus said this:

Then the King will say to those on his right, "Come, you who are blessed by my Father; take your inheritance, the kingdom prepared for you since the creation of the world. For I was hungry and you gave me something to eat, I was thirsty and you gave me something to drink, I was a stranger and you invited me in, I needed clothes and you clothed me, I was sick and you looked after me, I was in prison and you came to visit me."

> Then the righteous will answer him, "Lord, when did we see
> you hungry and feed you, or thirsty and give you something
> to drink? When did we see you a stranger and invite you in, or
> needing clothes and clothe you? When did we see you sick or in
> prison and go to visit you?"
>
> The King will reply, "Truly I tell you, whatever you did for one
> of the least of these brothers and sisters of mine, you did for me."
> (Matthew 25: 34–40)

As you restore your temple completely you will have more to give. More time, more love, more compassion. You will have more awareness and more energy. More health and more stamina. Most important, you will have more of Jesus. As you learn to build your relationship with Him, your cup will overflow in many ways, which will be of great benefit also to those around you.

Rest for your soul and worship of our God is the last building block of your restoration plan. It is not by chance that we end with worship of our Creator. He is the cornerstone of this restoration plan. His truths are woven throughout each building block. It is therefore fitting that we end with time to reflect and worship Him. It is the only possible reaction to the sense of awe and appreciation you should feel for the way He is restoring your life.

Conclusion

*Do you not know that in a race all the runners run,
but only one gets the prize? Run in such a way as to
get the prize. Everyone who competes in the games
goes into strict training. They do it to get a crown
that will not last, but we do it to get a crown that
will last forever. Therefore I do not run like someone
running aimlessly; I do not fight like a boxer beating
the air. No, I strike a blow to my body and make it
my slave so that after I have preached to others,
I myself will not be disqualified for the prize.*
1 CORINTHIANS *9:24–27*

You are now equipped with the information and tools you need to begin the lifelong process of restoring your temple. As Paul said in Corinthians, this is a race. You will need self-discipline for this strict training. The prize will make it worth it. So worth it.

You may ask, "What is the prize?" There are many prizes. Health, stamina, and physical fitness are some of them. Improved relationships and prioritization of your time are others. You will have an overall sense of well-being and achievement. All of these things will surely result from your commitment to this project. However, this only scratches the surface.

The ultimate prize Paul talked about is also within your grasp: you will gain a new or improved relationship with your Father and Creator. You will not be disqualified. He wants to know you and will reveal Himself to you through this. You will gain security and peace through Him. You may just secure the most amazing prize of all: eternal life with Him.

It says in Revelation 3:20, *"Here I am! I stand at the door and knock. If anyone hears my voice and opens the door, I will come in and eat with that person, and they with me."* This is your invitation. Jesus is patiently knocking at your door. The most important decision you will ever make (if you have not done so already) is to let Him in. He wants to know you fully. He wants you to know Him and His will for your life completely. I will say it again because it is so awesome: the Creator God of the universe wants in to your life to build a loving relationship with you. What are you waiting for?

Your restoration begins now!

What If I Am Not a Christian?
What If I Am Not Sure?

L et's start with this: God loves you and wants a relationship with you. There is no better time to start pursuing that than right now. How do you do this? It starts with a decision and then becomes what you spend the rest of your life entering into.

You may ask, "What is the decision and how do I make it?" Let's see what the Bible has to say about this.

- *"If you declare with your mouth, 'Jesus is Lord,' and believe in your heart that God raised him from the dead, you will be saved"* (Romans 10:9).
- *"Jesus replied, 'Very truly I tell you, no one can see the kingdom of God unless they are born again'"* (John 3:3).
- *"When the disciples heard this, they were greatly astonished and asked, 'Who then can be saved?' Jesus looked at them and said, 'With man this is impossible, but with God all things are possible.'"* (Matthew 19:25–26).

So in summary, this is not something you can accomplish on your own. You can however, through Jesus, gain eternity with God and a personal relationship with Him. You do this by:

- Saying with your mouth that "Jesus is Lord."

- Believing with your heart that God is who He is, and that the Bible truly teaches us what He did.
- Letting your life be a testimony to these beliefs through obedience to His Word and abiding in God in good times and tough times.

Here is a prayer you could say to begin this relationship with the loving, all-knowing, and all-powerful God of your life.

> God, I know I need to start living my life for You and with You. I have been living for myself but recognize I need You. Please be in my life and help me to obediently walk on the path You have created for me. I acknowledge that Jesus Christ is God and died for me on the cross, and I want the forgiveness You give me as a gift through this loving and necessary sacrifice. Enter my life completely. Be my God and Father. Be my Rock and Redeemer. Be my Teacher and Guide. You are the Truth and the Way. I will no longer be controlled by sin and the desires of this life. I will live my life to follow You. Guide me in this with your grace and mercy. I ask this in Jesus's name. Amen.

Welcome home.

Part II

WEEKLY WORKSHEETS

Week 1

Building Block 1 Prayer and Study: Prepare Your Soul and Mind

- Start every day with prayer followed by silent time with God.
  S___ M___ T___ W___ T___ F___ S___
- Read this week's readings (see appendix). Each time ask, "What does this reading say?" and "What does it mean for me?"
- How is God speaking to you through His Word?

Building Block 2 Diet: Fuel Your Body

- Keep the ten rules handy until you know them well.
- Refer to the lists in the appendix often.
- Learn the foods on the shopping list and plan meals and recipes that use them. Try the grilled avocado recipe.
- Keep track of these recipes (especially the ones that you like).
- Track these at least three days this week:
  Carbs (g)   S___ M___ T___ W___ T___ F___ S___
  Sugar (g)   S___ M___ T___ W___ T___ F___ S___
  Fat %   S___ M___ T___ W___ T___ F___ S___
- Rate your current overall health and satisfaction with your weight from 1-100: _____

Building Block 3 Exercise: Strengthen Your Temple

- Thirty minutes per day for three to six days (put an X to keep track—you need three to six X's total)
  Strength   ___ ___ ___
  Stamina   ___ ___ ___
  Flexibility   ___ ___ ___
- Start strong and be committed to this.

Building Block 4 Stress Reduction: Find Peace for Your Soul

- Hand over one of your stressors to the Lord in prayer this week
- Write in your prayer journal at least 5 nights this week (optimal goal = every night)
  S__ M__ T__ W__ T__ F__ S__
- Answer these three questions in your prayer journal:

- What three things are you thankful for today?
- In what way did you best restore your temple today?
- How did you see God work in your life today?
- Use music to find some peace. This week's song recommendations: "God's Not Dead" by Newsboys and "Start a Fire" by Unspoken.

Building Block 5 Community: Choose Your Companions

- Learn the hierarchy of your relationships
- Make sure you are not spending more time on your phone, computer, or television than you are spending doing one of the following three things:
  - Time in prayer or study (Building Block 1)
  - Time exercising (Building Block 3)
  - Time in community with those at the top of your hierarchy list (Building Block 5)
- Is there a relationship that comes to mind needing your immediate time or attention?

Building Block 6 Removing Toxins: Cleanse Your Life

- If you smoke and have not stopped already, now is the time.
- Use EWG.org to replace some toxic chemicals in your home with safe alternatives
- Consider starting with a more natural deodorant

Building Block 7 Rest and Worship: Reset Your Compass

- Do you feel rested from your sleep?
- Consider using a sleep tracker
- Put an X if you woke up feeling rested:
  S___ M___ T___ W___ T___ F___ S___
- Attend worship this week and answer the four questions from this chapter in regard to the place of worship.
- Enjoy a day of rest

Bible Readings

- Isaiah 9:6–7
- Matthew 1:18–25
- Matthew 2
- Luke 2:1–40
- Matthew 3
- John 2:1–25

Week 2

Building Block 1 Prayer and Study: Prepare Your Soul and Mind
- Start every day with prayer followed by silent time with God.
  S___ M___ T___ W___ T___ F___ S___
- Read this week's readings (see appendix). Each time ask, "What does this reading say?" and "What does it mean for me?"
- How is God speaking to you through His Word?

Building Block 2 Diet: Fuel Your Body
- Keep the ten rules handy until you know them well.
- Refer to the lists in the appendix often.
- Learn the foods on the shopping list and make meals and recipes using them. Try the barbacoa recipe.
- Track these at least three days this week:
  Carbs (g)   S___ M___ T___ W___ T___ F___ S___
  Sugar (g)   S___ M___ T___ W___ T___ F___ S___
  Fat %   S___ M___ T___ W___ T___ F___ S___
- Are you seeing or feeling any changes?

Building Block 3 Exercise: Strengthen Your Temple
- Thirty minutes per day for three to six days (put an X to keep track—you need three to six X's total)
  Strength   ___ ___ ___
  Stamina   ___ ___ ___
  Flexibility ___ ___ ___
- Are you sore? Fight through it.

Building Block 4 Stress Reduction: Find Peace for Your Soul
- He is listening. Tell Him what is on your mind.
- Write in your prayer journal at least five nights this week (optimal goal = every night)
  S__ M__ T__ W__ T__ F__ S__
- Answer these three questions in your prayer journal:
  - What three things are you thankful for today?
  - In what way did you best restore your temple today?

- How did you see God work in your life today?
- Use music to find some peace. This week's song recommendations: "Fix My Eyes" by For King & Country and "Everything" by Lighthouse

Building Block 5   Community: Choose Your Companions

- Be aware of and restore the hierarchy of your relationships.
- Make sure you are not spending more time on your phone, computer, or televisions than you are spending doing one of the following three things:
  - Time in prayer or study (Building Block 1)
  - Time exercising (Building Block 3)
  - Time in community with those at the top of your hierarchy list (Building Block 5)
- Are you surrounding yourself with Christian friends—those who will help and be supportive to you?

Building Block 6   Removing Toxins: Cleanse Your Life

- Use EWG.org to replace some toxic chemicals in your home with safe alternatives. This week look at your dish soap and detergent.

Building Block 7   Rest and Worship: Reset Your Compass

- Do you feel rested from your sleep?
- Consider using a sleep tracker.
- Put an X if you woke up feeling rested:
  S___ M___ T___ W___ T___ F___ S___
- Attend worship this week and answer the four questions in regard to the place of worship.
- Enjoy a day of rest.
- Give of your time or resources to someone in need.

Bible Readings

- Mark 1:14–45
- Mark 2:1–17
- Matthew 4
- Matthew 5
- Matthew 6

Week 3

Building Block 1   Prayer and Study: Prepare Your Soul and Mind

- Start every day with prayer followed by silent time with God.
  S___ M___ T___ W___ T___ F___ S___
- Read this week's readings (see appendix). Each time ask, "What does this reading say?" and "What does it mean for me?"
- How is God speaking to you through His word?

Building Block 2   Diet: Fuel Your Body

- Stay strong this week! Try the Anti-inflammatory Green Smoothie.
- Track these at least three days this week:
  Carbs (g)   S___ M___ T___ W___ T___ F___ S___
  Sugar (g)   S___ M___ T___ W___ T___ F___ S___
  Fat %   S___ M___ T___ W___ T___ F___ S___

Building Block 3   Exercise: Strengthen Your Temple

- Thirty minutes per day for three to six days (put an X to keep track—you need three to six X's total)
  Strength   ___ ___ ___
  Stamina   ___ ___ ___
  Flexibility   ___ ___ ___

Building Block 4   Stress Reduction: Find Peace for Your Soul

- Write in your prayer journal at least 5 nights (optimal goal = every night)
  S__ M__ T__ W__ T__ F__ S__
- -Answer these 3 questions in your prayer journal:
  1. List three things you are thankful for today.
  2. In what way did you best restore your temple today?
  3. How did you see God work in your life today?
- -Use music to find some peace - Song Recommendations: "7 * 70" by Chris August and "How He Loves" by John Mark McMillan.
- -Did you go to the Lord during a stressful time this week?

Building Block 5   Community: Choose Your Companions

- -Be aware of and continue to focus on the hierarchy of your relationships.

- -Make sure you are not spending more time on your phone, computer, or televisions than you are spending doing one of the following three things:
  - Time in prayer or study (Building Block 1)
  - Time exercising (Building Block 3)
  - Time in community with those at the top of your hierarchy list (Building Block 5)
- Is there someone in your life you need to forgive? This is the week to do it.

Building Block 6 Removing Toxins: Cleanse Your Life

- Use EWG.org to replace some toxic chemicals in your home with safe alternatives. How about your shampoo and body soap?

Building Block 7 Rest and Worship: Reset Your Compass

- Do you feel rested from your sleep?
- Put an X if you woke up feeling rested:
  S___ M___ T___ W___ T___ F___ S___
- Attend worship this week.
- Enjoy a day of rest.
- Give of your time or resources to someone in need.

Bible Readings

- Mark 6:14–56
- Luke 13:10–17
- Luke 4:1-14
- Mark 12
- John 9

Week 4

Building Block 1 Prayer and Study: Prepare Your Soul and Mind
- Start every day with prayer followed by silent time with God.
  S___ M___ T___ W___ T___ F___ S___
- Read this week's readings (see appendix). Each time ask, "What does this reading say?" and "What does it mean for me?"
- How is God speaking to you through His word?

Building Block 2 Diet: Fuel Your Body
- Do not weigh or measure yourself until next week at the earliest.
- Track the following on one day this week:
  Carbs (g) S___ M___ T___ W___ T___ F___ S___
  Sugar (g) S___ M___ T___ W___ T___ F___ S___
  Fat %   S___ M___ T___ W___ T___ F___ S___
- Rate your current overall health and happiness with your body from 1-100: _____
- If you had a day where you ate something outside of the rules. How did you feel? Write about it in your journal.
- Try the Apple-Basil Chicken Burgers with the sweet potato slices.

Building Block 3 Exercise: Strengthen Your Temple
- Thirty minutes per day for three to six days (put an X to keep track—you need three to six X's total)
  Strength   ___ ___ ___
  Stamina   ___ ___ ___
  Flexibility ___ ___ ___
- Are you feeling stronger?

Building Block 4 Stress Reduction: Find Peace for Your Soul
- Write in your prayer journal at least five nights (optimal goal = every night)
  S__ M__ T__ W__ T__ F__ S__
- Answer these three questions in your prayer journal:
  - What three things are you thankful for today?
  - In what way did you best restore your temple today?

- How did you see God work in your life today?
- Use music to find some peace. This week's song recommendations: "10,000 Reasons" by Matt Redman and "I Am" by Crowder.

Building Block 5   Community: Choose Your Companions

- Be aware of and restore the hierarchy of your relationships, focusing this week on your spouse.
- Make sure you are not spending more time on your phone, computer, or televisions than you are spending doing one of the following three things:
  - Time in prayer or study (Building Block 1)
  - Time exercising (Building Block 3)
  - Time in community with those at the top of our hierarchy list (Building Block 5)
- Start planning a weekly or biweekly date night with your spouse.

Building Block 6   Removing Toxins: Cleanse Your Life

- Use EWG.org to replace some toxic chemicals in your home with safe alternatives.
- Have any mental or thought toxins plagued you this week? Talk about this in your prayer time and/or with a trusted Christian friend or family member.
- Consider the use of essential oils. Try the inhaler recipe.

Building Block 7   Rest and Worship: Reset Your Compass

- Do you feel rested from your sleep?
- Attend worship this week. Is God speaking to you?
- Enjoy a day of rest.

Bible Readings

- John 10
- John 11
- Luke 9
- Luke 10
- Luke 22:1–6

Week 5

Building Block 1   Prayer and Study: Prepare Your Soul and Mind
- Start every day with prayer followed by silent time with God.
  S___ M___ T___ W___ T___ F___ S___
- Read this week's readings (see appendix). Each time ask, "What does this reading say?" and "What does it mean for me?"
- How is God speaking to you through His word?

Building Block 2   Diet: Fuel Your Body
- Track (optional this week):
  Carbs (g)   S___ M___ T___ W___ T___ F___ S___
  Sugar (g)   S___ M___ T___ W___ T___ F___ S___
  Fat %   S___ M___ T___ W___ T___ F___ S___
- Record your weight and any other measurements you would like to track here:
  Weight:_____
  Waist size:_____
  Other measurements:_____

Building Block 3   Exercise: Strengthen Your Temple
- Thirty minutes per day for three to six days (put an X to keep track—you need three to six X's total)
  Strength   ___ ___ ___
  Stamina   ___ ___ ___
  Flexibility   ___ ___ ___

Building Block 4   Stress Reduction: Find Peace for Your Soul
- Write in your prayer journal at least five nights (optimal goal = every night)
  S__ M__ T__ W__ T__ F__ S__
- Answer these three questions in your prayer journal:
  - What three things are you thankful for today?
  - In what way did you best restore your temple today?
  - How did you see God work in your life today?

- Use music to find some peace. This week's song recommendations: "Everything Glorious" by David Crowder Band and "By Your Side: by Tenth Avenue North.

Building Block 5   Community: Choose Your Companions

- Be aware of and maintain the hierarchy of your relationships.
- Make sure you are not spending more time on your phone, computer, or televisions than you are spending doing one of the following three things:
  - Time in prayer or study (Building Block 1)
  - Time exercising (Building Block 3)
  - Time in community with those at the top of our hierarchy list (Building Block 5)
- Are you being present (not thinking about something else or looking at your phone) during conversations?

Building Block 6   Removing Toxins: Cleanse Your Life

- Use EWG.org to replace some toxic chemicals in your home with safe alternatives.
- Evaluate some of your other cleaning supplies.

Building Block 7   Rest and Worship: Reset Your Compass

- Do you feel rested from your sleep?
- Put an X if you woke up feeling rested.
  S___ M___ T___ W___ T___ F___ S___
- Attend worship this week.
- Enjoy a day of rest.
- Give of your time or resources.
- Is there anything in your life you feel God calling you to change or think deeply about?

Bible Readings

- John 12:1–19
- Luke 22:7–38
- Mark 14:32–72
- Luke 23:26–43
- John 19:28–42

Week 6

Building Block 1 Prayer and Study: Prepare Your Soul and Mind

- Start every day with prayer followed by silent time with God.
  S___ M___ T___ W___ T___ F___ S___
- Read this week's readings (see appendix). Each time ask, "What does this reading say?" and "What does it mean for me?"
- How is God speaking to you through His word?

Building Block 2 Diet: Fuel Your Body

- Track the following on one day this week:
  Carbs (g) S___ M___ T___ W___ T___ F___ S___
  Sugar (g) S___ M___ T___ W___ T___ F___ S___
  Fat %   S___ M___ T___ W___ T___ F___ S___
- Is there anyone else you know who would benefit from this?

Building Block 3 Exercise: Strengthen Your Temple

- Thirty minutes per day for three to six days (put an X to keep track—you need three to six X's total)
  Strength   ___ ___ ___
  Stamina   ___ ___ ___
  Flexibility ___ ___ ___
- What have been the benefits of consistent exercise for you? How will you maintain this for the rest of your life?

Building Block 4 Stress Reduction: Find Peace for Your Soul

- Write in your prayer journal at least five nights (optimal goal = every night)
  S__ M__ T__ W__ T__ F__ S__
- Answer these three questions in your prayer journal:
  - What three things are you thankful for today?
  - In what way did you best restore your temple today?
  - How did you see God work in your life today?
- Use music to find some peace. This week's song recommendations: "Beautiful Mystery" by 513 Free and "More of You" by Colton Dixon.

- Any stressors this week you need to pray about and hand over to the Lord?

Building Block 5   Community: Choose Your Companions

- Be aware of and continue to focus on the hierarchy of your relationships.
- Spend some quality, focused time with each of your children.
- Make sure you are not spending more time on your phone, computer, or televisions than you are spending doing one of the following three things:
  - Time in prayer or study (Building Block 1)
  - Time exercising (Building Block 3)
  - Time in community with those at the top of our hierarchy list (Building Block 5)
- Can you go this whole week without social media? I dare you to try.

Building Block 6   Removing Toxins: Cleanse Your Life

- Use EWG.org to replace some toxic chemicals in your home with safe alternatives. Check out your cosmetics.

Building Block 7   Rest and Worship: Reset Your Compass

- Do you feel rested from your sleep?
- Attend worship this week.
- Enjoy a day of rest.
- Give of your time or resources.

Bible Readings

- John 20
- John 21
- Acts 9
- 1 Corinthians 15
- Revelation 3:20

Week 7

Building Block 1 Prayer and Study: Prepare Your Soul and Mind
- Start every day with prayer followed by silent time with God.
  S___ M___ T___ W___ T___ F___ S___
- Read this week's readings (see appendix). Each time ask, "What does this reading say?" and "What does it mean for me?"
- How is God speaking to you through His word?

Building Block 2 Diet: Fuel Your Body
- No need to track this week!
- If you had a recent day where you ate something outside of the rules. How did you feel? Write about it in your journal.
- Record your weight and any other measurements you would like to track here:
  Weight:_____
  Waist size:_____
  Other measurements:_____
- Could you guide someone else to eat this way? Who would it be?

Building Block 3 Exercise: Strengthen Your Temple
- Thirty minutes per day for three to six days (put an X to keep track—you need three to six X's total)
  Strength   ___ ___ ___
  Stamina   ___ ___ ___
  Flexibility ___ ___ ___
- This is just the beginning. You made it seven weeks. Now it is a habit.

Building Block 4 Stress Reduction: Find Peace for Your Soul
- Write in your prayer journal at least five nights (optimal goal = every night)
  S__ M__ T__ W__ T__ F__ S__
- Answer these three questions in your prayer journal:
  - What three things are you thankful for today?
  - In what way did you best restore your temple today?

- How did you see God work in your life today?
- Use music to find some peace. This week's song recommendations: "Build Your Kingdom Here" by Rend Collective and "How Can It Be" by Lauren Daigle.

Building Block 5   Community: Choose Your Companions

- Be aware of and restore the hierarchy of your relationships.
- Make sure you are not spending more time on your phone, computer, or televisions than you are spending doing one of the following three things:
  - Time in prayer or study (Building Block 1)
  - Time exercising (Building Block 3)
  - Time in community with those at the top of our hierarchy list (Building Block 5)
- Is there someone who comes to mind you could mentor?
- Strongly consider starting a regular time of fellowship or small group with other Christians.

Building Block 6   Removing Toxins: Cleanse Your Life

- Use EWG.org to replace some toxic chemicals in your home with safe alternatives.
- Consider using essential oils.

Building Block 7   Rest and Worship: Reset Your Compass

- Do you feel rested from your sleep?
- Attend worship this week.
- Give of your time or resources.
- Enjoy a day of rest and prepare to enjoy the rest of your life in relationship with the God who loves you. Plan to apply the principles learned in the last seven weeks for the rest of your life. Use this book as a guide.

Bible Readings

- James 1
- James 2
- James 3
- James 4
- James 5

Week 8 and Beyond

Building Block 1 Prayer and Study: Prepare Your Soul and Mind

- Start every day with prayer followed by silent time with God.
S___ M___ T___ W___ T___ F___ S___
- "To be a Christian without *prayer* is no more possible than to be alive without *breathing*." *Martin Luther*
- Continue studying God's word as a part of your life starting with reading one Proverb per day for the next month and then the Gospels (Matthew, Mark, Luke, and John) or a Bible study of your choosing.
- How is God speaking to you through His word?

Building Block 2 Diet: Fuel Your Body

- Remember the rules and stay strong in your new way of fueling your temple.
- Could you guide someone else to eat this way? Who would it be?

Building Block 3 Exercise: Strengthen Your Temple

- Thirty minutes per day for three to six days (put an X to keep track—you need three to six X's total)
Strength   ___ ___ ___
Stamina   ___ ___ ___
Flexibility   ___ ___ ___

Building Block 4 Stress Reduction: Find Peace for Your Soul

- Write in your prayer journal at least five nights (optimal goal = every night)
S__ M__ T__ W__ T__ F__ S__
- Answer these three questions in your prayer journal:
  - What three things are you thankful for today?
  - In what way did you best restore your temple today?
  - How did you see God work in your life today?
- Use Christian music to find some peace and for worship.

Building Block 5   Community: Choose Your Companions

- Be aware of and restore the hierarchy of your relationships.
- Make sure you are not spending more time on your phone, computer, or televisions than you are spending doing one of the following three things:
  - Time in prayer or study (Building Block 1)
  - Time exercising (Building Block 3)
  - Time in community with those at the top of our hierarchy list (Building Block 5)
- Strongly consider starting a regular time of fellowship or small group with other Christians.

Building Block 6   Removing Toxins: Cleanse Your Life

- Use EWG.org to replace some toxic chemicals in your home with safe alternatives.
- Consider using essential oils.

Building Block 7   Rest and Worship: Reset Your Compass

- Do you feel rested from your sleep?
- Attend worship this week.
- Give of your time or resources.
- Enjoy a day of rest.

NEXT STEP!!!

Christianity starts with a loving, obedient, and personal relationship with God, but that is the beginning, not the end. We are called to pass it on, to be fishers of men. So my challenge to you is this: **mentor someone else through seven weeks of Restore Your Temple.** It could be someone who came to mind during your seven week journey or someone who has been asking about it. It could be multiple people. I hope this book can serve as your tool to spread the good news. It is your turn to shepherd someone in their walk. In medical school there is a saying, "see one, do one, teach one". This is how we learn best. It is your turn to be the teacher now that you are moving along the *narrow path*. Remember, we are called to love one another. Is there any better way to love someone than to walk with them towards Jesus?

Appendix

Diet Rules
Shopping List
Dirty Dozen
MSG List
Names for Sugar
A Day of Eating for Me
Exercise Plan
Prayer
Hierarchy of Relationships
A Few Recipes
Aromatherapy

Diet Rules

There is a more detailed version in Building Block 2.

- Limit added sugar to near elimination. You should consume less than thirty grams per day and less than five grams per serving.
- Remove MSG and other chemically altered ingredients from your diet.
- Remove gluten from your diet. Your maximum grams of other carbs per day should be 150g.
- Limit dairy, except cultured organic butter or ghee.
- Most of your diet should consist of one-ingredient foods from the shopping list.
- Limit alcohol.
- Don't count calories.
- Eat lots of healthy fat and organic or grass-fed proteins.
- Eat lots of vegetables.
- Eat three servings of God-created fruits (not juice).

The Shopping List

It is time to go shopping and to start to seriously think about how and what you are going to eat. Let's start with a shopping list. The list will have five categories:

- Protein/meat
- Vegetables
- Fruit
- Fats
- Other

Here is a Temple Restoration Plan version of a food pyramid:

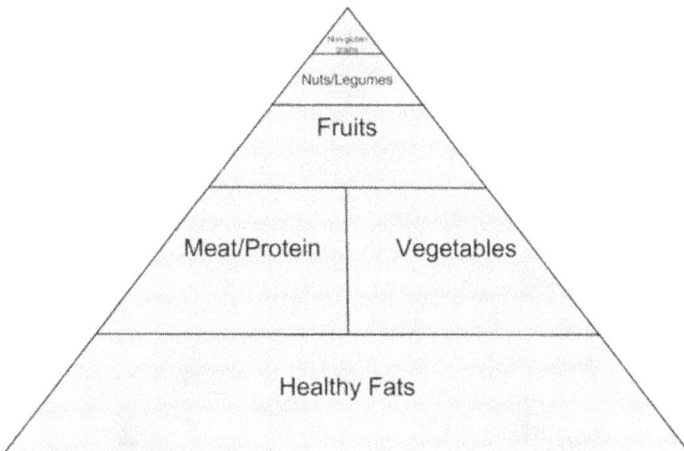

Protein/Meats

<u>Optimal</u>
Grass-fed or organic beef (or buffalo, elk, venison, lamb)
Pasture-raised or organic chicken
Wild-caught seafood
Pasture-raised, organic eggs
Pasture-raised or organic pork

<u>Good</u>
Lean, trimmed store-bought beef, chicken, pork, lamb
Regular store-bought or omega-3 eggs

<u>Limited</u> (unless none of the added ingredients break any of the ten rules)
Processed meats such as bacon, sausage, deli meats

Vegetables

Optimal
Avocado
Acorn squash
Arugula
Asparagus
Broccoli
Bok choy
Brussels sprouts
Butternut squash
Cauliflower
Collard
Cabbage
Cucumber
Kale
Olive
Leek
Shallot
Sweet potato and yam
Zucchini

Good
Beet
Bell pepper
Carrot
Celery
Eggplant
Green bean
Onion
Peas
Pumpkin
Mushroom
Radish
Rutabaga
Rhubarb
Snap pea
Spaghetti squash
Summer squash
Sprouts
Tomato
Green onion
Lettuce
Watercress

Limited
Corn
Potato

Fruits

Optimal

Blackberry
Blueberry
Grapefruit
Coconut
Strawberry
Raspberry
Lemon and lime
Cranberry
Pineapple

Good

Apricot
Apple
Banana
Cantaloupe
Cherry
Fig and plum
Grapes
Kiwi
Mango
Melon
Orange
Clementine
Tangerine
Pomegranate
Watermelon
Peach
Pear
Plum
Melon (other)
Papaya
Guava
Passion Fruit

Limited

Dried Fruit
Jams and Jellies
Canned Fruit

Fats

<u>Optimal</u>
Extra-virgin coconut oil
Extra-virgin olive oil
Cultured grass-fed, organic butter
Ghee
Avocado oil

<u>Limited</u>
Regular butter

<u>Do Not Eat</u>
Margarine, spreads, vegetable oil, canola oil, most other oils

Other

Nuts and Seeds
These are for occasional consumption. They should have minimal ingredients with no artificial additives (other than maybe a little sea salt). Most flavored nuts and seeds have off-limits ingredients and oils.

<u>Optimal</u>
Almond
Cashew
Hazelnut
Pecan
Macadamia
Pistachio
Walnuts (or their butters, without added sugars)
Most seeds

Legumes
One to two servings per day is allowed and may be beneficial. Check your ingredients—no additives allowed.

<u>Optimal</u>
Kidney
Black
White
Red
Chick peas
Lentil

<u>Limited</u>
Peanut
Peanut Butter

<u>Do Not Eat</u>
Soybean

Grains
Other carbohydrates like oats (eat gluten-free only), rice, buckwheat, amaranth, and quinoa should be used on a somewhat limited basis and

preferably at dinner. They should not be the main course or source of calories. Non-gluten grains such as coconut or almond flour can also be used. Gluten is off limits. As a goal, keep total carbohydrates below 150 mg per day.

Spices

One-ingredient spices are allowed, and many are beneficial to your health. Have fun with them. But check the ingredients on all of your spices. Especially watch for spice mixes and powders, as most have additives. Experiment with making your own "safe" mixes. For example, instead of using a garlic salt mix, use garlic powder and a little sea salt.

Apple cider vinegar is allowed, as is organic 100 percent cacao powder.

Sweeteners

All of these should be limited to occasional use.

Xylitol (from American hardwoods, not corn) or Stevia as an alternative to sugar

Organic honey

Chocolate (try 90 percent dark chocolate or chocolate chips by Enjoy Life).

Beverages

Water is of course your main source. Your goal should be about half your body weight in ounces per day. For example, 150 pounds means about seventy-five ounces per day. An important indicator of a well-hydrated body is your urine, which should be light yellow rather than dark or clear.

Coffee and tea are allowed as long as what you are adding to it fits into the rules. Butter, ghee, and coconut oil are delicious in coffee. Limited amounts of almond or coconut milk are also acceptable if you watch for added sugar and other ingredients.

Not allowed are sodas (including diet), sports drinks, soy milk, juice, or any drink with added sugar.

Supplements

I will keep it simple and just tell you what I take (and recommend):

- 2000 IU Vitamin D per day (especially in the northern states where sunlight may be limited)
- 240 mg R-Lipoic Acid per day
- 350 mg Magnesium per day (try Natural Calm brand)
- Occasional probiotic

Just make sure to check your capsules and pills for additives (use plant-based capsules).

Dirty Dozen: Buy These Organic

- Apples
- Strawberries
- Grapes
- Celery
- Peaches
- Spinach
- Bell Peppers
- Nectarines
- Cucumbers
- Cherry Tomatoes
- Snap Peas
- Potatoes

Names of Ingredients Containing Processed Free Glutamic Acid (MSG and MSG-like additives)

More than forty different ingredients contain the chemical in monosodium glutamate (processed free glutamic acid). The following is a list of ingredients which contain processed free glutamic acid. It has been compiled over the last twenty years from information provided by manufacturers and food technologists.

Ingredients that *always* contain processed free glutamic acid:
- Glutamic acid
- Glutamate
- Monosodium glutamate
- Monopotassium glutamate
- Calcium glutamate
- Monoammonium glutamate
- Magnesium glutamate
- Natrium glutamate
- Yeast extract
- Anything "hydrolyzed"
- Any "hydrolyzed protein"
- Calcium caseinate
- Sodium caseinate
- Yeast food
- Yeast nutrient
- Autolyzed yeast (extract)
- Modified food starch
- Textured protein
- Soy protein
- Soy protein isolate
- Vetsin
- Ajinomoto
- Disodium 5'-guanylate
- Disodium 5'-inosinate
- Disodium 5'-ribonucleotides

Ingredients that *often* contain processed free glutamic acid:

- Carrageenan
- Bouillon and broth stock
- Flavors or flavoring
- Maltodextrin
- Anything ultra-pasteurized
- Barley malt
- Protease
- Anything enzyme-modified
- Anything containing enzymes
- Malt extract
- Soy sauce
- Soy sauce extract
- Anything protein-fortified
- Anything fermented
- Gelatin
- Whey protein
- Whey protein concentrate
- Whey protein isolate

Adapted from Truth in Labelling.[10]

Common Names for Sugar on Food Labels

- Anhydrous dextrose
- Brown sugar
- Confectioner's powdered sugar
- Corn syrup
- Corn syrup solids
- Dextrose
- Fructose
- High-fructose corn syrup (HFCS)
- Honey
- Invert sugar
- Lactose
- Malt syrup
- Maltose
- Maple syrup
- Molasses
- Nectars (e.g., peach nectar, pear nectar)
- pancake syrup
- Raw sugar
- Sucrose
- Sugar
- White granulated sugar

"A Day in My Life" Diet

Breakfast: Bulletproof® Coffee

- 10 oz. coffee from (fresh ground USDA organic beans) blended with:
  - 1 Tbsp. of Organic Ghee
  - 1 Tbsp. of Brain Octane™ Oil
  - 1 tsp of organic %100 cacao
  - Vitamin D, R-Lipoic Acid

Lunch: My "1-2-3 Lunch"

- 1 Organic apple
- 2 Clementines
- 3 Hard-boiled eggs

Dinner

- 1.5 organic chicken breasts
- 0.75 cup brown rice
- 1 cup cooked organic baby carrots
- 1 cup cooked broccoli
- 1.5 Tbsp. olive oil
- 1 Tbsp. coconut oil
- 0.5 cup black beans
- 1 Tbsp. grass-fed organic butter

Anti-Inflammatory Green Smoothie (sometimes with lunch or breakfast)

1 cup organic baby spinach
1 cup organic baby carrots
1 Avocado
1 organic apple
3/4 cup unsweetened organic coconut milk
2 Tbsp. lime juice
1 Tbsp. of Brain Octane Oil
1 Tbsp. olive oil

Bedtime

Chamomile tea with added Natural Calm magnesium supplement

Overall this is approximately:
- less than 150 grams of carbohydrates
- sixty grams of sugars, which are almost entirely from God-made fruit (far less than thirty grams from added sugar)
- 65 percent of the calories from fat

My 7-Week Workout Plan

All workouts are from Beachbody PiYo or P90X3. (I am not a Beachbody coach.)

Week	Day 1	Day 2	Day 3	Day 4	Day 5	Day 6	Day 7
1	PiYo Sweat	CVX	PiYo Core	Total synergistics	The Challenge	Off	Off
2	PiYo Drench	Incinerator	P90X3 Ab Ripper	Eccentric upper	The Warrior	Off	Off
3	PiYo Sweat	MMX	PiYo Core	Total synergistics	The Challenge	Off	Off
4	PiYo Drench	Incinerator	P90X3 Ab Ripper	Eccentric upper	Eccentric lower	Off	Off
5	PiYo Sweat	The Warrior	PiYo Core	Total synergistics	The Challenge	Off	Off
6	PiYo Drench	Incinerator	P90X3 Ab Ripper	Eccentric upper	Eccentric lower	Off	Off
7	PiYo Sweat	MMX	PiYo Core	Total synergistics	The Challenge	Off	Off

General Workout Plan

Week	Day 1	Day 2	Day 3	Day 4	Day 5	Day 6	Day 7
1	Strength	Cardio	Strength	Core - Flexibility	Strength	Off	Off
2	Strength	Cardio	Strength	Core - Flexibility	Strength	Off	Off
3	Strength	Cardio	Strength	Core - Flexibility	Strength	Off	Off
4	Strength	Cardio	Strength	Core - Flexibility	Strength	Off	Off
5	Strength	Cardio	Strength	Core - Flexibility	Strength	Off	Off
6	Strength	Cardio	Strength	Core - Flexibility	Strength	Off	Off
7	Strength	Cardio	Strength	Core - Flexibility	Strength	Off	Off

Prayer: ACTS

ACTS of Prayer (How to Pray)

1. Adoration and Praise: "God, I adore you because you are . . ."

- Putting into words the gratitude we should have whenever we consider all that God has done for us. Thanking and praising God for who He is.

2. Confession: "God, I confess that I have . . ."

- *If we confess our sins, he is faithful and just and will forgive us our sins and purify us from all unrighteousness* (1 John 1:9).
- Be real with ourselves and with God about our shortcomings.
  - God won't answer our prayers when there is unconfessed sin in our lives.
  - God won't forgive us unless we forgive others (see Matthew 6:14–15).
  - Confession has an effect upon our physical health (see Psalm 32:3–7).
  - God is not against us because of our sin. He is with us against our sin.

3. Thanksgiving

- *Do not be anxious about anything, but in every situation, by prayer and petition, with thanksgiving, present your requests to God* (Philippians 4:6).
- Adoration vs. thanksgiving:
  - Adoration is thanking God for who He is.
  - Thanksgiving is thanking God for what He has done.
- We should give Him thanks in all things (see 1 Thessalonians 5:18).

4. Supplication (asking God to supply)

- Ask for personal requests. Especially:
  - Wisdom (see James 1:5–8)
  - Health (see 2 Corinthians 12:7–9)
  - Daily needs (see Matthew 6:33)
  - Resisting temptation (see Matthew 26:41)
- Pray for and present requests for others.

Hierarchy of Relationships

Our relationships should be structured as such:
1. God
2. Spouse (if married)
3. Your children
4. Parents
5. Extended family
6. Fellow Christians
7. Non-Christians

Relational Circles
You can also think of this concept as relational circles.

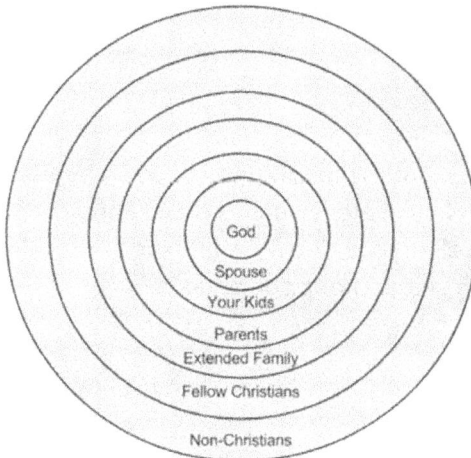

Recipes

Grilled Avocado with Chicken

Ingredients (serves 2)
  2 ripe, fresh avocados, seeded and peeled
  2 chicken breasts
  2 Tbsp fresh lime juice
  Olive oil
  Sea salt to taste
  Cumin
  Cilantro
  1/2 cup fresh chopped tomatoes or pico de gallo
  Fresh ground pepper to taste

Instructions

Grilled Avocado
  1. Cut avocado in half the long way and remove seed with a spoon.
  2. Drizzle with fresh lime juice and brush lightly with olive oil.
  3. Gently place cut side down on grill for 2 to 3 minutes.
  4. Season with salt and pepper to taste.

Grilled Chicken
1. Sprinkle chicken with olive oil, cumin, sea salt, and pepper (can also add garlic and/or cayenne pepper).
2. Grill chicken over medium heat.
3. Cut cooked chicken into small pieces and serve over grilled avocado half shells.
4. Can serve with chopped tomatoes or pico de gallo. Salsa is also an option if it is without unwanted additives.

Barbacoa

Ingredients
1 (2.5 to 4 pound) beef brisket
3 Chipotle peppers or chiles
2 cups of water
3 large cloves of garlic
2 tsp of oregano
1/2 tsp of ground cloves
1 Tbsp of apple cider vinegar
2 bay leaves

Instructions
1. Put chipotle peppers or peppers, water, garlic, oregano, cloves, apple cider vinegar, and bay leaves into blender. Blend to a puree/liquid.
2. Pour 1/4 of the liquid puree into the bottom of a slow cooker.
3. Trim any excess fat from the brisket and place it in your slow cooker with the fatty side down.
4. Pour the rest of the liquid puree over the brisket coating the top and sides.
5. Cook on low for 8 hours.
6. Remove the brisket and pull/shred with 2 forks. The brisket should pull easily.
7. Serve with vegetables or potentially 1/2 cup of cooked brown rice seasoned with butter.

Green Anti-Inflammatory Smoothie

Ingredients
    1 organic apple
    1 peeled avocado, pit removed
    Handful of organic spinach
    Handful of baby carrots
    1 cup organic coconut milk (ingredients coconut and water)
    1 Tbsp olive oil
    1 Tbsp of Bulletproof Upgraded Brain Octane Oil or Coconut Oil
    1/2 cup of water
    Few cubes of ice

Instructions
    1. Put everything in a blender and blend until smooth to liquid consistency.
    2. Add more water during the blending process if necessary.

Apple-Basil Chicken burgers

Ingredients (makes 6 burgers)
    • 1.5 lbs. ground chicken
    • 2 eggs
    • 1/2 cup coconut flour
    • 1/2 tsp salt
    • 1/2 tsp pepper
    • 1 red bell pepper, finely chopped
    • 1 apple, peeled and chopped
    • 3 Tbsp basil

Instructions
    1. Mix all the ingredients together
    2. Form 5 to 6 patties
    3. Heat coconut oil in a frying pan
    4. Cook the burgers on medium heat for 10 minutes on each side

Baked Sweet Potato Slices

Ingredients
- 2 large sweet potatoes
- 2 Tbsp olive oil or melted coconut oil
- 2 tsp dried rosemary
- 1 tsp sea salt

Instructions
1. Preheat oven to 375 degrees F.
2. Peel sweet potatoes and cut into thin slices (a Salad Shooter works well).
3. In a large bowl, toss the sweet potatoes with olive oil (or coconut oil), rosemary, and salt.
4. Place sweet potato slices in a single layer on a baking sheet covered with foil or parchment paper.
5. Bake for 15 to 20 minutes or until they start to brown.

Aromatherapy

Quick supply list for a kick start
- Lavender 100 percent essential oil
- Sweet Orange 100 percent essential oil

Make a Hand Sanitizer

What you will need:
2-ounce flip-top bottle
Aloe Vera gel
Grain or rubbing alcohol
Lavender, Eucalyptus, Geranium, Bergamot or Tea Tree essential oils

How to:
- Add one ounce of aloe vera gel to bottle
- Add one ounce grain or rubbing alcohol
- Add 10 drops of two oils of your choice (20 drops total).
- Shake well and use liberally.

Make Your Own Aromatherapy Inhaler

What you will need:
Small container
Rock salt
Lavender Essential Oil
Orange Essential Oil

How to:
- Fill container half full with rock salt.
- Add 2 to 4 drops of lavender oil.
- Add 3 to 5 drops of orange oil.
- Inhale as needed.

Room Spray

What you will need:
    2-ounce bottle
    Lavender, Eucalyptus, and Bergamot (or Orange) essential oils

How to:
- Add water to a two-ounce bottle, allow a bit of room.
- Add ten drops each of eucalyptus, lavender, and bergamot oil.
- Shake well before misting. Avoid spraying over varnished wood. Use as often as desired.

Endnotes

1 *Fed Up*. 2014. DVD. Stephanie Soechtig.

2 America's Health Rankings,. 2015. '2014 - Americas Health Rankings Report - State Health Statistics Brought To You By Americashealthrankings.Org.'. http://www.americashealthrankings.org/.

3 NPR.org,. 2011. 'How Western Diets Are Making The World Sick'. http://www.npr.org/2011/03/24/132745785/how-western-diets-are-making-the-world-sick.

4 National Center for Health Statistics (US). Health, United States, 2008: With Special Feature on the Health of Young Adults. Hyattsville (MD): National Center for Health Statistics (US); 2009 Mar. Chartbook. Available from: http://www.ncbi.nlm.nih.gov/books/NBK19623/

5 Connecticut College. "Are Oreos addictive? Research says yes." ScienceDaily. www.sciencedaily.com/releases/2013/10/131015123341.htm.

6 Wheatbelly.com Wheat Belly FAQs – Wheatbelly. 2015. 'Wheat Belly Faqs - Wheatbelly'. Accessed March 3, 2015. http://www.wheatbelly.com/articles/WBFAQs.

7 https://www.bulletproofexec.com/how-to-make-your-coffee-bulletproof-and-your-morning-too/

8 http://www.apa.org,. 2013. 'Stress In America 2013 Highlights: Are Teens Adopting Adults' Stress Habits'. http://www.apa.org/news/press/releases/stress/2013/highlights.aspx.

9 Emarketer.com,. 2013. 'Social Usage Involves More Platforms, More Often - Emarketer'. http://www.emarketer.com/Article/Social-Usage-Involves-More-Platforms-More-Often/1010019.

10 http://www.truthinlabeling.org/hiddensources.html.